Improving Nursing Performance Using a System Approach to Measurement

Timothy P. Williams and Mary E. Geary

Precept Press, Chicago
Division of Bonus Books, Inc.

01 00 99 98 97   5 4 3 2 1

Library of Congress Cataloging-in-Publication Data

Williams, Timothy P.
    Improving nursing performance using a system approach to measurement / Timothy P. Williams and Mary E. Geary.
        p.   cm.
    Includes bibliographical references and index.
    ISBN 0-944496-56-3 (alk. paper)
    1. Nursing audit.   2. System analysis.   I. Geary, Mary E.
    [DNLM: 1. Nursing Audit—methods.   2. Nursing Care.   WY 100.5   W727i   1997]
RT85.5.W575   1997
362.1'73'0685—dc21
DNLM/DLC
for Library of Congress   97-23917
                                                                  CIP

Precept Press
Division of Bonus Books, Inc.
160 East Illinois Street
Chicago, Illinois 60611

Table of Contents

To Melissa, Nicholas,
Laura and Patrick

Introduction

This text has been prepared to give the professional nurse an introduction to Performance Improvement (PI). The text follows a progression from theoretical principles to practical application of systems analysis and measurement. It is our intent that you will be able to apply these principles to real life situations.

The text is divided into three distinct sections. The first section describes the management theory that supports PI, provides the foundation of a nursing application of PI and introduces you to the PI style of nursing management. Section two discusses practical application, tools of implementation, data management, and transition from traditional nursing quality activities to PI. Section three focuses on practical application of nursing involvement in accreditation and using information management systems.

We hope that this book will be used by practicing nurses, students, and teams that are called upon to implement PI in their organization. A glossary of the most common words used in the PI environment is included to enhance your vocabulary. Read the first section thoroughly so that you are completely familiar with PI history and techniques. Even readers who are familiar with PI will find it useful to review this material so that concepts are completely understood. Without this basic background, a foundation for the practical application of PI will be a difficult undertaking. When you are comfortable with your knowledge of PI, section two will link the theory of PI to the reality of nursing practice. Read it carefully: a different approach to nursing management is outlined with PI and system/process thinking as the driving force. Gather together in teams within your organization and apply the tools, principles, and techniques of PI to real life situations. To properly demonstrate collaborative nursing practice, the PI approach will greatly enhance systems thinking and data-driven decision making.

Here are several initial assumptions:

1. You are a student nurse, staff nurse, nurse manager, or nursing leader.
2. You have been advised to read this book because your organization has embraced the PI approach to quality.
3. You are not satisfied with the "status quo" and are looking for a better way to conduct business.
4. You are willing to strive for the highest possible level of service to your ultimate customer—the patient.

Actually, whoever you are, and whatever you do, the information in this book will set you on the right course to PI in the workplace. As you will see, PI is not new. The struggle lies in involving all disciplines in a collaborative approach to measuring process function and working together on areas to improve. Nursing transition and involvement in PI has been slow and, at times, painful.

The lack of responsible, coordinated, and purposeful actions by professional nurses contributed to spiraling medical costs, inadequate staffing, low morale, and low pay. Emphasis on the clinical component of nursing practice is not enough. Health care is a business. A big business. Long-term and short-term goals and decisions must be based in fact. Measurement and analysis of appropriate systems/processes is the answer.

Statistical methodologies are an integral part of the PI philosophy. Other industries rely on statistics as the backbone of their business and decision-making. Payers in health care are an example of one enterprise deeply entrenched in statistics. If they couldn't predict a member's risk of illness or accident accurately, the business would soon fail.

Health care professionals deal with people. And people, as you know, come in all shapes and varieties. They do, however, tend to respond to a given action with some predictability. It is this predictability that forms the basis of PI

Transferring PI concepts from theory to practice, may seem difficult. Yet, PI's basic principles can be easily understood. With this understanding, application of the Performance Improvement philosophy in health care can readily be made.

Our goal is to provide a framework within the practice of nursing to transition nurses from traditional thinkers in quality concepts to collaborative systems thinkers. Data and facts will become your allies. Turning these data and facts into useful information will be your challenge. If knowledge is power, and information is knowledge, then understanding the principles in this text are essential for nursing practice.

Timothy P. Williams

Mary E. Geary

1

Performance Improvement Defined

Performance Improvement in health care has evolved over the past years, changing in definition and emphasis. Twenty years ago, quality assessment departments consisted of a few employees, usually nurses, who audited patient charts for signatures and correct forms. Because these activities did not necessarily influence quality of care, "quality assurance" programs were established with the assumption that quality care already existed and that data just needed to be collected to show that practice and outcomes were 100 percent effective. Nursing Quality Assurance (QA) flourished in organizations across the country and "unit based QA" programs abounded. Committees and members eagerly collected data on aspects and indicators of care. However, this process emphasized quantity, not quality. Soon all efforts focused on collecting data with little consideration of quality. Although the intent of the quality assurance efforts was estimable, many aspects of the program failed to improve outcomes of care.

A large amount of data was gathered, but few nurses possessed skills to analyze the data. As a result, QA committees did not know when or how to take improvement actions. In addition, because we were striving for perfection the areas of practice being monitored were found to be 100 percent, indicating no need for improvement. Areas of outcomes or practice that were performing at less than 100 percent were often not monitored for fear of punishment because deficits were believed to be caused by people. Nursing QA was dreaded by many managers. If one department showed more deficits than another, that department was negatively perceived.

Employees or other departments were usually blamed, clouding any attempts to focus on an issue and identify needed changes.

The structure of QA programs within organizations also contributed to program ineffectiveness. Each department looked at outcomes independently of other departments, although delivery of patient care is not isolated in one department or area. Thus, improvement in care was impossible because entire processes were never examined. For example, the QA committee in the Physical Therapy department monitored the number of patients arriving late for their treatment from other areas of the hospital. Because the PT department was not involved in preparing and transporting patients to PT, they were unable to improve this outcome independently. As long as this problem was monitored in isolation of the rest of the departments involved, it would never be solved. A similar situation occurred when the nursing department monitored the timeliness of STAT medications. Until the entire process was reviewed, including the pharmacy's role in preparing the medication, improvement could not be achieved.

QA programs evolved into Quality Improvement (QI) programs once leaders began to view their organization as an entire system. Adopting a "systems thinking" approach transformed quality efforts from being fragmented and departmentalized into being accurate measures of organizational performance. This change from QA to QI was influenced by many factors, including Total Quality Management (TQM), the management philosophy that had been so successful in much of the business world, and the Joint Commission on Accreditation of Healthcare Organizations' "Agenda for Change," which revised how organizations were surveyed for accreditation. Both of these factors are foundations for Performance Improvement programs today.

TQM PRINCIPLES

There are several prominent players in the TQM field. Each, not surprisingly, has his own definition of quality.

Dr. Joseph M. Juran

Juran defines quality as "fitness for use." He states that there must be freedom from deficiencies, such as number of defects, number of errors, hours of rework, and cost of poor quality. The product or service must also meet the customer's perceived needs. Juran further outlines his trilogy for quality improvement.

I. Quality Planning
  — Identify customers
  — Identify customer needs
  — Develop product features that respond to customers' needs
  — Develop processes that are able to produce those product features

II. Quality Control
  — Evaluate actual quality performance
  — Compare quality performance to quality goals
  — Act on the difference

III. Quality Improvement
  — Develop the infrastructure needed to secure annual quality improvement
  — Identify the specific needs for improvement
  —For each project establish a Project Team with clear responsibility for bringing the project to a successful conclusion.
  —Provide resources, motivation, and training needed by the teams to diagnose the cause, to determine the remedy, and to establish controls to hold the gains.

Dr. W. Edwards Deming

Deming defines quality as "continually meeting customers' needs and expectations at a price they are willing to pay." Deming expands on this definition with his fourteen points which are featured later in the book. The "Seven Deadly Diseases" is a list of common problems that impede Performance Improvement in non-TQM organizations. Deming's obstacles to transformation to TQM are also vital to Performance Improvement.

Deming's Seven Deadly Diseases

1. Lack of constancy of purpose to develop the product or service that will have a market and keep the company in business, thus creating more jobs.
2. Emphasis on short-term profits; short-term thinking (opposite of constancy of purpose to stay in business) fed by fear of an unfriendly takeover, and by a push from bankers and owners for dividends.
3. Personal review system, or evaluation of performance, merit rating, annual review, or annual appraisal, for people in management. Management by objective, on a go, no-go basis without a method for accomplishing the objective.
4. Mobility of management, or job-hopping.

5. Use of visible figures only for management with little or no consideration of the lesser known.
6. Excessive medical costs.
7. Excessive liability costs fueled by lawyers who work on contingency fees.

Deming's Obstacles to Transformation

1. Neglect of long-range planning and transformation.

    You hear it often: "There's no time to do this now, I've got to handle another problem." Leaders often get caught up in the "survival mentality" when, most of the time, these "problems" are more perceived than real.

2. The supposition that solving problems with automation, gadgets, and new machinery will transform industry.

    Avoid relying on technology to manage the business. Resist the computer company's sales pitch that promises more productivity and efficiency. Today's popular computers are not capable of fulfilling those promises entirely.

3. Searching for examples.

    Instead of looking for examples to solve your problems, look for reasons why another organization is successful.

4. Assuming your problems are different.

    While no two organizations are the same, it is possible to have similar problems. The excuse that your problems are in some way unique is most often wrong.

5. Obsolescence in schools (of business).

    Schools of business management still work on outdated theories of management by results.

6. Reliance on quality control departments.

    It is unreasonable to assume that the quality assurance staff is solely responsible for verifying quality standards. Providing a quality service is everyone's responsiblity.

7. Blaming the work force for problems.

    Management often shifts the blame away from the system, which, according to Deming, is responsible for 85 percent of the problems.

8. Quality by inspection.

    Change your thinking from looking only at outcomes to also focusing on the process.

9. False starts.

    A false start occurs when a company embraces only a part of the TQM philosophy. Training all employees in statistical methods, unsupported by the other components, will not work, according to Deming. False starts contribute to the "Here comes another one of the boss' big ideas" syndrome.

10. The unmanned computer.

    There are many types of unmanned computers. One type is the computer that holds huge chunks of meaningless data that is never used. Another is the computer that is used most often to make computer signs or party invitations.

11. Meeting specifications.

    When an organization is content to merely meet specifications, quality improvement is impossible.

12. Inadequate testing of prototypes.

    The demand to get a product or program to the public overshadows the need to make sure it works well.

13. "Anyone who tries to help us must understand everything about our business."

    Deming, a statistician, has clients from all possible business arenas. The basic tenets of TQM can be applied to all facets of the service industry—even nursing.

Phillip Crosby

Crosby defines TQM as a strategic, integrated management system for achieving customer satisfaction that involves all managers and employees and uses quantitative methods to continuously improve an organization's processes. The goal is to meet customer requirements. Much of the Crosby theory follows the basic concepts of general systems theory, input . . . throughput . . . output, with a feedback mechanism for improvement. Crosby says the process of work takes place in the throughput section.

This theory is described in what Crosby calls the absolutes of TQM. These include: quality (conformance to requirements), system (prevention), personal performance standard (do it right the first time), and measurement (price of non-conformance or zero defects). The application of zero defects in health care is difficult.

The Crosby approach to TQM comes from the aerospace industry and is heavily influenced by quality control concepts. Its application to health care is yet to be adequately tested. The concept of zero defects, when dealing with the human element is, in and of itself, nearly an impossible notion.

JCAHO Agenda for Change

The Joint Commission on Accreditation of Healthcare Organizations (JCAHO) has long since been a strong influence in health care quality programs. As part of its survey criteria, JCAHO has defined standards of quality. Its primary mission is to improve the quality of care provided to the public. It once had a separate chapter for quality activities which primarily required meeting a minimum standard of care. However, the JCAHO leaders realized that one quality department could not affect the overall quality of an entire organization, and improving performance should be the ultimate goal. JCAHO began their "Agenda for Change" in 1986; currently, Joint Commission Standards reflect a systems thinking approach which emphasizes quality in all functions and processes within the health care organization.

Many TQM concepts are reflected in the JCAHO approach to improving health care, including customer expectations, systematic design and redesign, measurement systems to measure processes and outcomes, and data analysis. Systems theory guides the survey process for total performance as an integrated system. All departments are viewed as working together to affect overall performance, patient outcomes, and quality of care. Instead of measuring departments separately, standards are now divided into functions with specific overall goals. Each function consists of many processes which involve many departments. For example, "Patient Assessment" is influenced by a variety of departments and staff. Nursing's patient assessment depends on input from the admitting department, laboratory, radiology, the physician, and others. Each department may have independent functions, but each influences the efficiency and effectiveness of performance. Emphasis is placed on improving performance of these processes when an opportunity for improvement exists.

Our Definition of Quality

The term quality has been given many definitions, each with its own merit. What quality means to one, it may not mean to another. From a total quality management perspective, the perception of the customer is paramount. In health care, there is another dimension to quality—standards. Standards do not always please the customer (patient), but they may be necessary to produce a positive outcome for the patient. An injection of penicillin in the buttocks may meet a standard and be the treatment of choice, but the patient may perceive the situation differently. Our definition of quality, as it relates to health care, must encompass both the customer's perception and standards.

Quality is both the customer's perception of the product or service provided and the supplier's knowledge of customer requirements, variation between customers, and applicable standards of practice.

Performance Improvement within an organization must also encompass the customer's perception of the care received and the standards of practice. This is accomplished by making goals and outcomes of each function and process reflect these quality components. In addition to patient perception and standards, there are basic PI components to build in to your PI program.

Basic Performance Improvement
Components

PI is not difficult to acheive once the basic tenets are understood. Common to all PI programs are the following basic components:

Customers

People or other organizations that use your services, including patients, families, physicians, employers.

Suppliers

People or companies that supply your needs, including physicians, nurses, payers.

Continuous Improvement

To stay competitive and to add value to your service, a continuous improvement philosophy must be in place. Continuous improvement means always striving for state-of-the-art products and services.

Corporate Culture

"We the people, in order to form a more perfect union . . . do ordain the Acme Vision Statement." Just as the U.S. Constitution set the vision for our country's corporate culture, an institution must set the vision for its corporate culture. The entire organization must strive for continuous Performance Improvement in quality of care. The outcomes of service and care are everyone's responsibility and are affected by the performance of systems within the organization.

Customers, suppliers, continuous improvement and corporate culture are four powerful concepts that will positively change the way an organization conducts business. The rest of this section explains PI as a management principle. We recommend reading and discussing its content with fellow workers, students, or colleagues.

2

Performance Improvement as a Management Principle

General Overview

It is important to distinguish Performance Improvement from Quality Assurance. They are very different. PI is an organizational philosophy and work culture which is shared by all. PI includes many TQM "tools," some which are concrete, such as bar charts, flow sheets, and forms, while others are abstract. The intangible tools are hidden within the system's thinking of PI and are more difficult to grasp.

QA, on the other hand, is not an organization-wide philosophy. Instead, it is a fragmented, departmental program designed to evaluate individual clinical practice. This evaluation can become *part* of your Performance Improvement efforts and serve as a building block for the transition to systems-wide PI. Quality based on inspection is not profitable for either the supplier or the customer. QA is not designed to be an inspection tool, although it was used by most organizations to find the bad apples and make quick fixes. QA was developed, rather, for one main purpose: to make an organization publicly accountable to the recipient of care or service. Traditional components of QA encompass four basic areas:

1. Privileging or competency;
2. Utilization management;
3. Risk management;
4. Monitoring and evaluation.

Each of these components will be described briefly so you will gain both a basic understanding of the difference between QA and PI and see how QA is a building block for a Performance Improvement process.

Privileging or Competency

Practitioners and providers of health care services must demonstrate that they are proficient, knowledgeable, and capable of providing appropriate services. This is accomplished in today's health care environment through a process of checks, validations, and licensing in each state and within every organization. Without appropriate credentials, the provider does not have a legal work permit to provide care or service to the patient. In the PI organization, quality care involves securing the right person to provide the right service the first time. Systems can only deliver quality outcomes if competent personnel are carrying out the appropriate functions.

Utilization Management

Utilization management (UM) involves the cost of care, or the cost of quality. The term cost of quality describes both the UM function as it pertains to QA, and the PI notion of spending resource dollars to improve care. UM in QA is an examination of the over, under, and optimum utilization of resources. Resources are simply defined as manpower, money, and machines. UM evaluates practice patterns to facilitate the delivery of low cost, efficient, and effective care to all patients. Components of a UM program include discharge planning, monitoring over/under utilization, identifying potential quality of care problems, and liability issues. These UM activities compliment a PI program as systems and processes needing improvement are identified.

Risk Management

Risk management (RM) involves protecting the liability of the organization while making the environment safe for patients, visitors, and staff. In today's health care arena, RM has taken on a preventive or prospective approach. The prudent risk manager is always examining and tracking data to identify high risk areas and procedures. Much of the data gathered in the QA mode are quality control monitors which directly relate to RM, such as medication errors, patient falls, and other incidents. In the Performance Improvement organization, constant system evaluation for improvement is the foundation of the RM process.

Monitoring and Evaluation

This component of QA involves actual evaluation of clinical practice. Through a system of standards and evaluation tools, data are gathered and analyzed to determine whether the providers of care and service are practicing adequately, or if there is need for improvement. QA began with monitoring and evaluating aspects of care within separate departments and on a case by case basis. As cases of poor quality were identified, they would be handled individually. Trending of data identifying the quantity of these "poor" instances of care was accomplished. But no system-wide approach to dealing with these cases was implemented. The PI model embraces an organization-wide approach to dealing with individual cases of poor quality of care. PI moves beyond simple inspection of provider performance and includes a review of processes within the hospital that support care and service.

The following principles embody the major components of PI.

Performance Improvement Principles

Top Management's Accountability

Today, when something goes wrong within a company, the CEO should feel the heat, not the worker. Top management is accountable for all processes and for the quality of those processes.

For example, the newborn nursery in one large urban hospital was experiencing a chronic problem with inadequate stock levels of small disposable diapers. The nurses were forced to use towels when the diaper supply was exhausted. Some of the newborns who were diapered developed moderate to severe perineal rashes and were forced to stay an extra day in the nursery before going home. The nurse manager made frequent calls to the supply department, but the response was sluggish.

In this case, the newborn nursery (customer) was not satisfied with the supply department (supplier). In a traditional organization, interdepartmental communication is difficult because individual departments are "disengaged" from each other. Lack of teamwork and cooperation leads to deficiencies in service. The hero in the traditional organization would probably be the irate middle level manager who copes with the shortage by storming into the supply department, confronting the supplier, and perhaps leaving with the diapers. Using this approach, the process never improved.

The PI organization would, by its very nature, have strong lines of communication and pre-established, supplier-customer relationships. The CEO must insist on a network that builds on company-wide PI. The nurse manager identifies a process which needs improving. Then, a PI team is formed to address the matter. In this example, three people (the nurse manager, a staff nurse, and a purchasing agent from the supply department) form the team that will review the current process and identify areas needing revision. Order lead times, stock levels, and diaper sizes would all be reviewed as part of this process. All work is a process and part of a larger system which strives to achieve the overall outcome: quality care. Clearly defined steps lead to the ultimate goal of providing such service.

Continuous Improvement Philosophy

The adage, "If it ain't broke, don't fix it," is the traditional approach to most processes. The PI health care facility goes one step further: "If it ain't broke, make it better." The goal is continuous improvement of service.

Deming's chain reaction best explains this: Improve quality—costs decrease because of less rework, fewer mistakes, fewer delays, better use of time and materials—productivity improves—capture the market with better quality and lower price—stay in business—provide jobs and more jobs.

A Performance Improvement framework allows an organization to continuously improve by acknowledging that no system is perfect. Rather than maintain the status quo, identify processes that can be redesigned for better performance and acknowledge that changes can create a productive atmosphere.

Customer-driven Organization

Recognize customer-supplier relationships within your organization. Patients, the ultimate customer, are always the priority. Patients can also be suppliers: they can supply feedback and suggestions—good and bad—for better service. Patients are known as external customers. Other external customers include the myriad of services that supply hospitals with what they need to conduct business.

Physicians are customers, too. In fact, next to patients, physicians are nurses' biggest customers. Establishing this customer-supplier relationship can help to smooth strained relationships in a hurry.

In any organization, you will find two types of customers—internal and external. Internal customers are found within the hospital. Each department or service is both a customer and a supplier of each other. The web of relationships seems complicated, but once mapped out and understood by all, getting the job done becomes much easier. The team approach greatly reduces the traditional barriers to communication and to understanding the role of each department. Performance Improvement teams, quality improvement teams, or process improvement teams—whatever you choose to call them—bring together staff members from all facets of the process in question.

If the team is built and nurtured correctly, members will have mutual respect and admiration for each other. This climate is developed through a variety of team building exercises and a common sense of purpose.

To illustrate how a small team would function, we will examine the need for diabetic patients to have their feet checked once a year by a podiatrist. The primary health care provider—a nurse practitioner in this case—needed to set up a straightforward approach to the relatively tedious process of routine foot exams with the podiatrist. The nurse practitioner simply visited the podiatrist, and together they drew up a simple protocol for the timing, pre-visit labs, and clinic hours. The nurse practitioner requested notification in writing of the results of the exam within a one-week period. They also agreed on standard patient educational material. This arrangement set in motion a very efficient process for preventing and detecting a tragic side effect of diabetes. The patients were delighted with the comprehensive care and the accessibility of the service. The podiatrist and nurse practitioner functioned as a team, complementing each other in their efforts to deliver quality care within their respective areas of expertise.

Service-Oriented Strategy

The customer must come first, last, and always. In nursing terms, this means quality patient care. Sadly, many organizations lose sight of this fundamental fact. Once they do, business suffers. For example, if a patron experiences slow service at a restaurant, chances are that he or she will quietly leave and not return. Further, he or she will probably discourage others from going there. Patients will seldom be upfront about their dissatisfaction with service. Constant feedback from your internal and external customer should be encouraged. Patient satisfaction surveys are excellent tools to identify opportunities for improvement from the customer's point of view. What patients perceive as quality care may be different from the supplier feels they need. People have different expectations and definitions of quality and the supplier must determine how well the organization is meeting their needs. In a recent study, Young et al., found that both nursing staff members and unit managers' beliefs regarding patient care values did not match those of their patients. Not understanding patient expectations of care may impede a hospital's attempts to improve customer reports of service quality.

New Management Style

Top management must work to convince and educate a critical mass of employees about Performance Improvement as the organizational culture. They must ensure that important processes of the organization are measured, addressed, and improved if possible. The critical mass in this case will be at least one-third of the organizational structure. Without the enthusiastic support of these people, significant Performance Improvement will be difficult. Resistance to change is a common problem. No one likes to upset the apple cart. Fear of losing jobs, suspicion, laziness, satisfaction with the status quo, and apathy are all characteristics of the difficult road to the transition. The literature in this area suggests that the transition toward the new corporate culture will take three to five years with numerous changes along the way. Some authors believe this transition can take from five to 10 years for some organizations. This long process is probably never complete because knowledge about improving processes and performance continues to evolve.

Work Force Empowerment

There are three main ingredients of work force empowerment. Natural participation is the first important component. There needs to be top to bottom involvement within the organization from the start. This means all levels must not only be educated in PI principles, but also must embrace the philosphy.

The second component of work force empowerment is influence without authority. Workers should become "process owners." Process ownership is a powerful motivator for the work force. Much like when an artist signs an oil painting, nurses must be able to put their name on what they do—and what goes on around them. People, in general, do not want to be robots: they want to be involved. This involvement includes the authority to influence these processes. Without this authority, the process is owned by a distant supervisor. In today's climate of constant change within the work place, it is important for nurses to feel they have control over their environment. Involvement in Performance Improvement activities provides this sense of control.

Some leaders resist workforce empowerment because they don't want to relinquish their power. Satisfaction with power will need to be replaced with the satisfaction of providing the best possible service. Job titles are what we've all been trained to strive for. In America, the only legal dictatorship appears to be the foreman—or the nurse manager. Therefore, the layers of management within the PI organization are necessarily "flattened," or consist of fewer levels.

The third component of work force empowerment is rewards. Reward employees based on quality-enhancing performance, not for "putting out fires" like traditional organizations do. Award employees for prevention-based activities instead of inspection or detection-based activities. Allow employees the freedom to say when a procedure is not working well, and allow them to be part of creating the solutions to improve the outcomes.

Prevention Oriented

The concept of prevention is easy to understand, but difficult to implement. The reasons for this are endless. Organic to any prevention effort is a strong planning focus. A Performance Improvement-based organization will plan a move carefully before implementing it. It is far less costly to fix the problem before it happens. A good rule of thumb for time line planning is to allow 90 percent for planning and 10 percent for implementation.

George S. Odiorne, in his book *The Change Resisters*, feels that Americans' optimism, their belief that everything will "turn out alright" precludes the need to plan. Events such as domestic terrorism, the end of the Cold War, and the more recent fall in our dominant economic power have prompted this country to plan better. Many people rely on luck and change to accomplish a task. This so-called anti-planning mentality is socially ingrained.

In a traditional American organization, planning is reserved for people who "play bureaucratic games" and are "stalling" against progress. Planning is not taken seriously. The annual plan is often called the "planning exercise." Health care organizations must change in today's economic environment. Serious efforts in planning and program design can result in changes for the better. Remember that failing to plan, or failing to plan seriously, is planning to fail.

Two types of planning are outlined:

Implicit planning is the free form style, similar to a "let's go and see what happens" Sunday drive. This isn't really planning at all. It's seat-of-the-pants impulse buying, freewheeling decisions based on mood or short-term experience with little forethought.

Explicit planning is a clearly thought-out plan which carefully considers all alternatives. Surprises, although possible, are held to a minimum. Unlike implicit planning, direction and purpose is instilled in every process. Implicit thinkers are living for the present moment and have only short-term goals, while the explicit planner studies past events in order to plan for the future.

The focus for leaders in health care organizations today should be on the planning stage in order to systematically improve performance. In a collaborative, interdisciplinary manner, an organization-wide plan for PI should be created, including prioritizing improvement activities. When a new process or service is designed, the mission and vision of the organization should be considered along with the needs and expectations of the customers. Efforts in up-front planning and design can make measurement, assessment, and improvement easier tasks in a systematic PI approach.

Team Approach

Teams should not be confused with committees. Committees are ordinarily a group of individuals who would rather be somewhere else, and exist largely due to policy requirement. On the other hand, teams consist of individuals desiring to work together to tackle a tough problem. This is PI's approach—carefully selected people getting together for the sole purpose of accomplishing a stated mission.

The team approach and team building strategies are important to master early. For more details on the team approach, see *The Team Handbook* by Peter S. Sholtes. It contains helpful information for those involved with project teams.

Statistical Thinking

As we will see in later sections, statistical thinking is involved in Performance Improvement. Statistical thinking is not foreign to nurses. Nurses always collect subjective and objective data during the evaluation phase. Consider the following:

1. *Management by the Facts*

Making decisions on known data is better than either guessing or "winging it." For example: Since the hospital began twelve-hour weekend shifts, medication errors have increased. Is it due to the extra long shift? The sample scatter diagram (Fig. 2-1) makes it clear that most of the medication errors do occur after the regular eight-hour shift. Armed with this

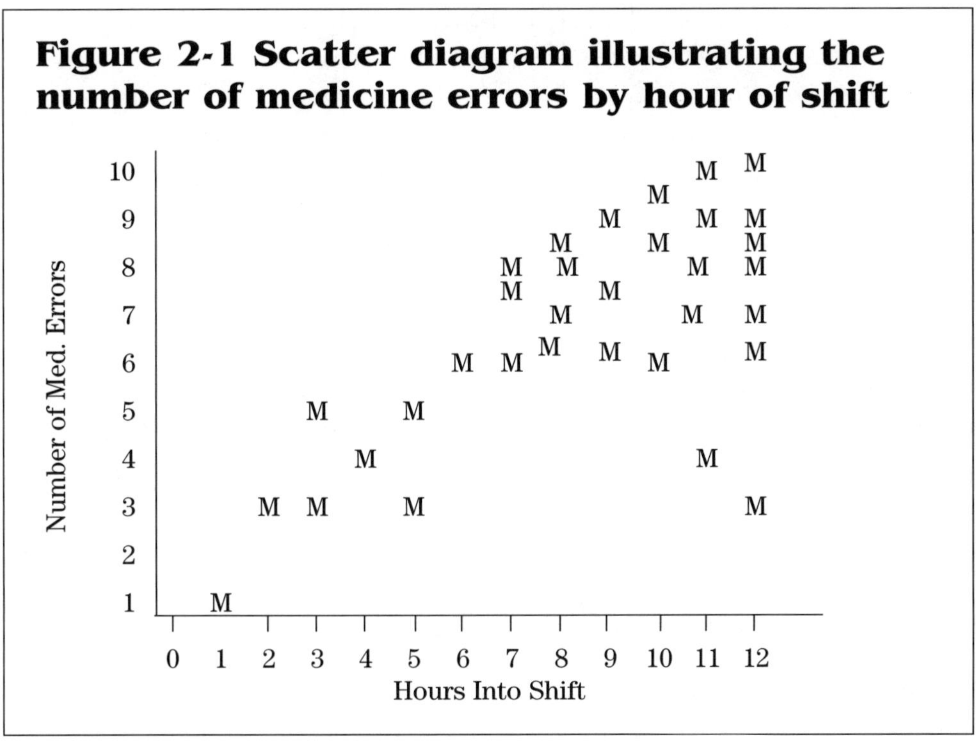

factual information, a Performance Improvement team works through a new system that is aimed at reducing medication errors.

2. *Orderly Approach*

Using the statistical tools to factually describe the process establishes a more orderly approach and leads to appropriate changes to improve performance.

3. *Benchmark*

The benchmark, or current statistical status, is an important concept. If the current status of many of your processes is unknown, then progress cannot be measured. Once an organization's status is determined, progress toward higher levels of quality can be measured. Comparing current performance with past performance is called internal benchmarking. Performance can also be compared with outcomes of similar outside organizations. Benchmarking uses measures of comparative performance to develop an understanding of how others have achieved higher levels of performance. There are many different definitions of benchmarking in health care today, but all of them have the following characteristics:

- Benchmarking is understood to be process, a structured approach, or a discipline.
- The process of benchmarking is continuous or ongoing.

- Benchmarking involves measuring, evaluating, and comparing both results and the processes that produce the results.
- Benchmarking focuses on the best practices and the best results.
- The goal of benchmarking is to document improvement.

Ongoing Education and Training

It is important for an organization to invest in its work force. This requires long-term commitment, including money and time, from top level management. Improving the worker will improve the quality of care, leading to increased levels of productivity and profit. This is best exemplified by the requirement for continuing education to maintain a nursing license.

Deming's "Fourteen Points"

Deming's fourteen points serve as a checklist for organizational quality improvement. The fourteen points will help organize the attempt to institute a performance improvement program.

Each of Deming's points deserves a chapter of in-depth analysis. It is beyond the scope of this book to describe each in detail. We recommend Mary Walton's book *The Deming Management Method* for more explanation. Listed below are the fourteen points and a brief explanation of each.

Point One: *Create constancy of purpose for the improvement of product and service*

Nurses need to examine their work habit: the process is at least as important as the outcome. Over time, the focus has shifted from the importance of the process to the outcome. PI falls somewhere in the middle. Nurses must engage in clinical research to refine the processes that bring positive outcomes. Redesigning traditional programs or establishing dramatically new programs may not be the answer. Efforts may be geared towards continually improving existing services and keeping the customer as our first priority.

Point Two: *Adopt the new philosophy*

Improving quality of service must become priority number one. Mistakes are beneficial because they are the stepping stones to improvement. This philosophy must be adopted by top management, and it must be pervasive within the organization. When patients feel they are central to service, an organization can be sure it has succeeded.

Deming's fourteen points, statistics, and team building are concepts easy to comprehend, but the transforming of the mind to this way of thinking may be difficult. Nurses need to become educated and socialized to their roles and responsibilities within the PI-based organization to be perceived as experts in their own right.

Point Three: *Cease dependence on mass inspection*

Finding the "bad apples" and blaming the worker, old QA, will not improve service. Deming states, "Quality comes not from inspection but from improvement of the process." Some advocates of PI feel that all inspection is bad, but sometimes inspection is justified—and necessary. Quality control measures of equipment functioning, medication, and infection control are regulated by inspection and are performed for safety reasons. An organization should ensure that inspection is carefully thought out, is cost effective, does not dominate the time and effort of the work force, and is understood to be a helpful tool, not a punishment.

Inspections according to certain specifications is absurd. There can be no improvement when the work is "alright" because it met a certain standard. Future performance should be considered. Improvements to meet future needs should be planned.

Point Four: *Do not award business on price tag alone*

This practice leads to major drawbacks. Ideally, an organization should use one supplier for a particular set of items and establish a long-term relationship. This will help to reduce paperwork and variation in the product, and will enhance customer-supplier relationships. Vendors will trust the organization more if they know they have a secure position with its customers.

Choosing the best supplier is not easy. A good supplier will deliver a high quality product and will accommodate any changes that need to be made along the way. Unfortunately, price tag lures many towards lower quality.

Point Five: *Constantly improve the system of production and service*

Performance Improvement is rooted in this principle. PI is a dynamic fluid state. Management must not be satisfied with the status quo, but should lead the way to improvement.

Avoiding the "zero defects" goal is important. The zero defects concept—that nothing ever goes wrong with the process—may work in some industries, but not in health care. This is an impossibility—especially when dealing with the human element of health care issues. A more realistic statement would be "We will reduce the variation, stay ahead of our competitors, and realize that each patient encounter is unique."

Point Six: *Institute training on the job*

Training, a natural extension of Performance Improvement, should be part of the work day. Develop training programs for all employees. Improper training is a system problem, not a person problem. The untrained or improperly trained worker often is blamed for a mistake that is really a system error. Eighty-five percent of all problems in an organization are probably system-process related. Some important questions to ask are: Is the person adequately trained for this job? Was enough time allotted for training? Is there a system of performance evaluation in place to ensure competency and correct technique and understanding of the job? How long has it been since this person was trained or evaluated on this task? Were requirements known or updated since the last training session?

Top management should invest heavily in its employees. Training not only improves the level of performance, it sends a message to the employees that they are valued and appreciated.

Training should be relevant to the job description. Workers at all levels will need training in Performance Improvement principles, basic statistical analysis, group dynamics, and problem solving techniques. Although workers may not use all the tools, everyone needs to know the basics. This involvement will foster both a sense of ownership in the organization and knowledge of the improvement process. The benefit is a worker with high morale.

Management should not allow the worker to train the worker. Similar to the telephone game, a simple message whispered down the line is often very different at the end. Provide a standard for training and follow the established standards. Your outcomes of training should be based on the following:

Typical Organizational Outcomes

Right Things Wrong	Right Things Right
Wrong Things Wrong	Wrong Things Right

Point Seven: *Institute leadership*

Leadership will facilitate Performance Improvement. It is essential that top management promotes improvement within the organization. Leaders should, among other things, be sensitive to employee perceptions. How an employee perceives his or her role is key. If the employee believes the boss wants the job done quickly, cheaply, or "as well as possible," the quality of service will suffer.

Some nurses have trouble collaborating with leadership. For some, the subservient role is deeply ingrained. Nurses harbor a wealth of vital information that never surfaces because they live either in fear of management or have low self-esteem. This is not to say that all nurses cower in the corner—nothing could be further from the truth. But, nurses should feel confident in their abilities and make an effort to contribute heavily to improving hospital procedures.

A leader does not have to be the CEO. The nurse manager or the staff nurse can be a leader. Deming advises leaders at all levels to know their employees' jobs, and to have a basic understanding of what they do.

Point Eight: *Drive out fear*

Fear in the work place is widespread and is manifested in many forms. It is at the core of what we do, say, and produce. To establish a work environment where Performance Improvement is possible, the employees must feel secure. Let's look at a secure situation.

In an ideal work place, nurses at all levels do not fear reprisal for their opinions or suggestions. In fact, suggestions are welcomed, and the leadership adopts many of them. Leaders are actively involved in training and development. Nurses are an active part of the problem-solving process and are, in fact, thought of as process owners. Fear among the work force is nonexistent. Suggestions for process improvement lead to higher quality.

Point Nine: *Break down barriers between staff areas*

"One hand doesn't know what the other is doing," is commonly heard in larger companies. In health care, it's especially difficult to be aware of all hospital activities because of the complexity of specialties and departments.

An organization should institute team work; build cross-functional, multidisciplinary teams to tackle Performance Improvement projects. In the traditional system of management, policy makers often force misguided policies into a system, then blame workers for not following directions when policies fail. Policy makers should not make decisions without staff input.

Point Ten: *Eliminate slogans, exhortations and targets for the work force*

"Do it right the first time!" "Zero Defects!" "There have been 365 days without an accident!" All are familiar slogans around the work place. Deming believes these only "generate frustration and resentment." There will always be mistakes, accidents, and defective materials. Although intended to inspire, these slogans do little else than set employees up for failure. Imagine working on a unit that had this sign on the nurses' locker room wall: "We have __ days without a needle stick!" This is like a time bomb. Management is asking for something it will never get—no needle sticks.

This example uses a number that grows with each passing day. Too many variables need to be considered when trying to prevent needle sticks.

Yet management holds you to this goal knowing that someday the number will return to zero. However, the number is not important! Relying solely on numerical goals for performance measurement is not realistic. Knowing *how* and *why* you succeed at any given task *is* realistic.

Point Eleven: *Eliminate numerical quotas*

Deming believes that quotas impede Performance Improvement more than any other working condition. Nurses don't have quotas like a piece worker who produces so many widgets per hour. Nurses have subliminal quotas. Get the report to the boss by nine—no matter what. Each nurse will care for 10 patients—regardless of their acuity.

The processes that contribute to common nursing pitfalls should be examined: why is a nurse who leaves the hospital on time thought to be a poor worker? The customer-first philosophy should persist. In this case, the customer is the nurse. The nurse may be tired or may have a family to get home to or simply have finished his or her responsibilities. Design a system which identifies, eliminates, and understands pitfalls. Ask nurses why they stay late. The answer is often, "There is no time during the day to chart patients." Top management and staff should look at why this is so. Does the unit have enough clerical support? Is the nursing staff adequate? Does the nurse need time management training?

Point Twelve: *Remove barriers to pride of workmanship*

Every nurse likes to feel appreciated, but sometimes nursing can be a thankless job. Emotions run high and burnout is common. As usual, the problem has many variables. Communication must be on the top of the list. Top management's duty includes listening to the people and giving them feedback. Possibly in no other profession is communication so vital.

Patients are a great source of praise. They give it often and are probably the reason nurses stay on the job. Supervisors should remove status barriers and management layers to allow improved interaction with their staff. This means working with the staff, not just dropping by to see how things are going. Leaders should have first hand experience with some of the frustrations of the workers so that they will be a in a better position to help solve those problems.

Point Thirteen: *Institute a vigorous personal program of education and self-improvement*

This point may seem obvious, but many organizations lack an effective training program. Some state nursing boards require a certain amount of continuing education—another quota, another numerical goal. This implies that once a specific goal is reached, the training is complete. Nothing could be further from the truth.

The medical field's knowledge base is changing at an increasing rate. Continuing education should be just that—continuing. Top leadership should invest in its workers and allow them to improve. Employees should be responsible for attending training sessions. An improved employee leads to improved performance. Hospitals that provide training, certification, and graduate degrees will have higher quality care, have a higher morale, and have more loyalty to the organization.

All nurses need to be educated in the simple statistical tools outlined in this book. Knowing how to think in this way will add one more person to the number of Performance Improvers.

An organization should establish and continually update the "corporate glossary." A strong vocabulary enhances the effectiveness of both communication and understanding. Performance Improvement, like almost everything else, has its own language. It is important for an organization to develop a comprehensive glossary. All companies should have the word "quality" in their glossary. Look at the two definitions below:

#1 Quality—We at Spacely Hospital believe that quality is doing your best with what you have.

#2 Quality—We at General Hospital believe that quality is our primary concern. Quality begins and ends with the customer. We are duty bound to our customers to provide the best possible service available anywhere in the world. To this end, we dedicate ourselves to increasing the quality of care.

The second definition is obviously more complete. Each organization's definition of quality will be different, but it should be easily understood by all employees.

Point Fourteen: *Take action to accomplish the transformation*

One of Deming's early mistakes in the U.S. was to concentrate on spreading the message of Performance Improvement to middle level management and below. Even though this group was impressed, Deming's methods never caught on. Top level executives were not convinced—perhaps because it wasn't their idea, or perhaps they didn't fully understand Deming's principles. Most importantly, Performance Improvement must start at the top level of management. The CEO and Nurse Executive must both adopt the new philosophy and disseminate it to the rest of the organization through education and involvement.

3

Performance Improvement Toolbox

Quality has been an abstract concept. Here, we hope Performance Improvement concepts will become tangible. This toolbox holds simple, yet powerful tools for persons involved in process improvement. Organizational leaders should know of these tools, but they often are not the originators of them. The members of a Performance Improvement team are responsible for creating these tools.

Many nurses shy away from research because they aren't comfortable with statistics. The tools in this chapter can be easily mastered. A calculator isn't necessary for most of them. Also, many different computer software programs can construct the different tools. Basic tools of Performance Improvement include brainstorming, Pareto charts, top-down flow charts, "Fishbone" diagrams, histograms, run sheets, and control charts. Other less used tools, such as the scatter diagram and the 25 cent tour, are also presented.

Before constructing the charts, some basic statistical concepts should be reviewed.

First Concept

All work can be either measured or counted. Some procedures are easily measured such as temperature, pulse, or respiration. What about an adverse medication reaction? It can't be measured, but it can be counted.

25

Second Concept

All work has a pattern, which is disclosed when analyzed using a check sheet and histogram. The normal shape—or distribution—will be like this: As illustrated in Figure 3-1, most of the data elements fall into the middle,

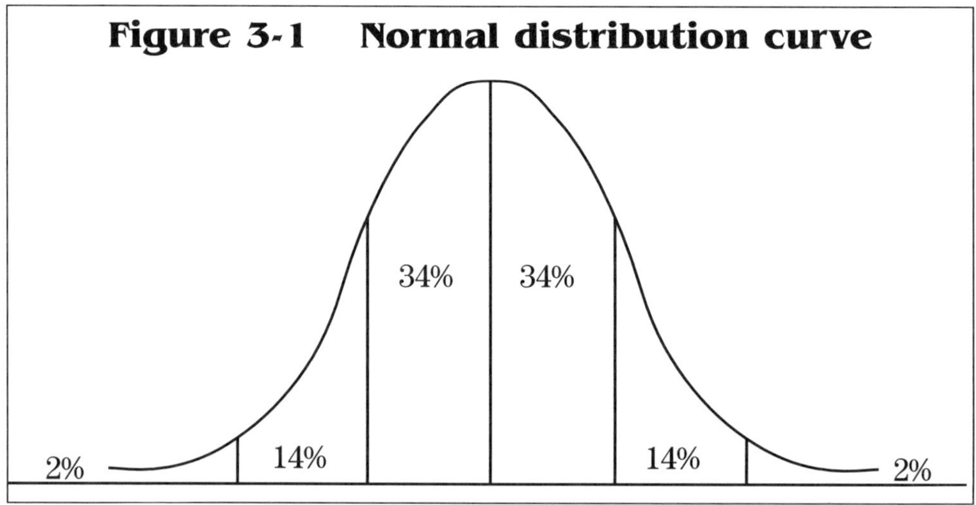

while very few fall within the "tails." Statisticians report that about 70 percent of all data fall within the middle two sections, 25 percent fall into the next two sections, and 5 percent fall into the remaining two sections. This knowledge can be applied to the next concept.

Third Concept

In any process, there is variation. Variation occurs because people are all different and will react differently to the same treatment modalities. However, there is an expected range of acceptable outcomes.

Example

Any lab result has a range of acceptable results. For the most part, the results will be within this range. This is called common cause variation. Special cause variation occurs when the lab result is outside the expected range. In the case of a lab result, such as a white blood cell count of 21,000, the special cause is most likely an infection somewhere in the body. A special cause variation needs special attention—probably antibiotics.

The concept of variation can be applied to other processes that do not involve the patient directly. There is variation in admission rates, nosocomial infections after surgery, readmission to a psych ward, or waiting time at the pharmacy for IV medications. All of these processes have variation. In the Performance Improvement organization, these variations would be measured. Common cause variations can be "narrowed" to a finely-honed machine. In the same fashion, special cause variations can be readily detected and acted on appropriately.

Situation Analysis—Team Building

A carpenter will tell you that you will need the right tools for the job. In Performance Improvement, there are many powerful tools to use, but it takes a certain knowledge to apply these tools correctly. The team approach is the most effective way to do this. So, before we explore the seven basic tools, let's take a look at the "toolbox" itself.

Performance Improvement is best accomplished with a group of people—a team who have a related interest and investment in the process in question. It is not fair to equate this group of persons to a traditional committee. The PI team is formed to improve the performance of a process, not to meet company standards or external regulations. Team members are asked to be on the team because of their knowledge and experience with the process being studied. Some key points in determining Performance Improvement team membership are:

1. Select a team leader who understands PI principles and techniques and can guide the team through its task.
2. Select a team facilitator familiar with group dynamics, team techniques, and PI principles.
3. Ensure adequate representation of all workers involved in carrying out the process being studied.
4. Select representatives from various job categories who have similar job functions.

The Nurse as a Team Member

Nurses crave teamwork. Historically, nurses have worked on various teams, acquiring different roles. Nurses are vital team members on many different hospital committees and task forces. Team involvement is not new to nurses. However, nurses may find participating on Performance Improvement teams a different experience and a welcome change from those of the past. Performance Improvement teams have one goal—an opportunity for improvement. The task is clear and the agenda is set. Members of the PI team were selected for the knowledge and expertise they bring to the process and the outcomes being examined. Everyone on the team is an active, participating member, in contrast to meetings that are run by one person and members are expected just to listen.

The PI team should meet with a clear purpose. This is different from the monthly mandatory committee meetings that nurses often dread and view as a waste of their time. Performance Improvement teams are work forces which create actions for improvement. Results can be seen which allow the nurse team member to feel productive, influential, and appreciated for his or her professional input.

Since PI teams are comprised of members from different departments (depending on the process being addressed), nurses are afforded the opportunity to work with other disciplines and professionals. As respect develops for each other's expertise and opinions, communication between departments and professionals is improved. Being a member on a PI team gives the nurse experience in systems thinking and problem solving, skills which are valuable tools in today's health care environment.

Empowerment

The concept of empowerment is central to effective team building. A seven step approach is outlined:

1. Assess the staff's competence and willingness to perform according to the job description (constancy of purpose).
2. Design an educational program tailored to the needs and wants of the staff (institute training).
3. Allow staff members to function autonomously after demonstrating competence. It is important for the nurse manager to emphasize this concept.
4. Provide support during the transition from dependent to independent practitioner (adopt a new philosophy). Use problem solving exercises to bolster confidence.
5. Clearly explain the risks that the new decision maker is taking. Be certain that the nurse is ready to assume these risks and understands the implication.
6. Ensure that staff nurses have communication skills that will support an expanded network of relationships. Let the staff know that the

leadership suports them, that it's acceptable to make mistakes, and that all situations need to be reported.

7. Institute the regular use of a team approach to problem solving. Education in group dynamics is necessary.

Empowerment is one of the "buzz words" of the nineties. It is a concept that can work well if it is implemented correctly. Following the aforementioned principles can help staff accept responsibility for their decisions and become independent thinkers. One hospital which did not establish the concept of empowerment evoked the following comment from a frustrated employee, "I have finally figured it out. The secret of empowerment is knowing when you are supposed to be empowered and when you aren't." In other words, inconsistency in management's philosophy of empowerment caused the staff to feel it was only a word on paper, not a concept to be followed. Empowerment, quite simply, is allowing employees to think on company time.

Tool Box

Basic Tools of Performance Improvement

I. TOOLS	II. TEAM ACTIVITIES	III. DATA ANALYSIS
BRAINSTORMING	25 CENT TOUR	PARETO CHART
STORY BOARDING	DATA COLLECTION	SCATTER DIAGRAM
NOMINAL GROUP	SURVEY TECHNIQUES	RUN CHART
TECHNIQUE	FOCUS GROUPS	CONTROL CHART
FISHBONE DIAGRAM	CHECK SHEETS	HISTOGRAM
TOP-DOWN FLOW CHART		
PROCESS FLOW CHART		

I. Tools

Brainstorming

Brainstorming is used to collect ideas from a group without regard to the validity of those ideas. This approach fosters creativity among group members if they can refrain from becoming judgmental during the brainstorming session. Sometimes what seems to be the craziest idea at the start is the best idea at the end of this process.

The rules are easy. Follow them carefully:

1. All group members have equal input into the process.
2. There should be no immediate discussion as to the validity of a suggestion. This comes later. There are no "dumb ideas." The wilder the idea the better. The purpose of brainstorming is to generate many ideas. The more ideas, the better chance of identifying the best one.
3. Appoint a leader to enforce the rules and a scribe to record the ideas.
4. When the group has finished suggesting, the ideas can be prioritized and addressed one at a time.

Brainstorming is an excellent method to uncover problems, suggest ideas, and enhance creativity. Choose a strong facilitator as "gate keeper" so the session does not get out of control. A word of caution: brainstorming may not be effective with a group of people who are unfamiliar with each other. Team members may not feel comfortable or may not trust other team members and may feel too threatened to say what is really on their mind. The leader should stress the rule that no idea is wrong, thus helping to promote input and participation.

Story Boarding

Story boarding is the midway point between brainstorming and the nominal group technique.

1. Team members anonymously write their ideas on an index card— one idea to a card.
2. The cards are given to the leader who reads all the ideas to the group.
3. With the help of the group, the ideas are placed on a board in pre-selected categories.
4. Once the ideas are sorted into categories, the group prioritizes each idea based on the project at hand.

Story boarding is an extremely effective way to elicit the best ideas from the group. It offers some anonymity, but still allows for group discussion regarding the relative weight of each idea. Any type of group can use this method. It is especially helpful, in early stages of PI teams, to examine issues and input from all members to determine all possible causes of variation. This type of exercise allows individuals to be honest in their responses.

Nominal Group Technique

The nominal group technique is useful when the project involves sensitive issues that require unpopular decisions. The steps in the nominal group technique include:

1. As in story boarding, all group members will anonymously write their ideas on an index card.
2. When the master list is created, the group will prioritize this list by secret ballot, usually listing the top three choices. Discussion can then be focused on the top contenders rather than on who suggested the ideas.

Fishbone Diagram

The fishbone or "cause and effect" diagram is attributed to Kaoru Ishikawa, a leading quality improvement authority in Japan. The effect, in this case, is the desired outcome, and the causes are the "spines." In its root form, the causes are generally divided into five basic categories: money, materials, methods, manpower, and machines. These categories can be amended to fit your topic. The following example demonstrates how this diagram can work.

You are the night nurse on a busy elective surgery unit. One of your biggest problems is that the pre-op lab slips are often not in the chart when the surgeon arrives for morning rounds. This has created much conflict among the nursing shifts and the surgeons. According to routine, the patient is instructed in a letter to come to the hospital for routine lab work the day before the surgery. Patients sometimes arrive the morning of surgery without having had the labs completed because they either forgot, didn't have time, didn't understand, or didn't bother to read the instructions. To make matters worse, the night lab staff cannot do some of the required labs because the machines are shut down in the evening for daily quality control. The unit secretaries are upset because when they come to work in the morning they are deluged with a myriad of lab slips to post. The secretaries claim they cannot complete the task of posting the lab slips and figuring out whose lab work is incomplete. This forces you to have the routine labs done on a STAT basis, which angers the lab staff. The surgeons arrive early expecting a completed chart and, of course, find them incomplete. They become angry with the day shift nursing staff for not preparing their patients "according to instructions" and delaying their surgery schedule. Sound familiar?

During a brainstorming session, a Performance Improvement team comprised of a representative from each nursing shift, a lab technician, a unit secretary, a patient, and a surgeon, identified many steps and barriers involved in the process. One helpful technique in identifying a problem is to ask why five times. Start with a general statement of one of the problems, then ask why it is so five times. Write down the answers for later reference.

For some patients, the labs are not ready in time for the surgery.

1. Why?
   Because the patients didn't come in ahead of time to have them done.
2. Why?
   Because they didn't understand the instructions.
3. Why?
   Because they couldn't understand the oral directions.
4. Why?
   Because the direction may be too complicated to understand.
5. Why?
   Because it is unreasonable to expect the patient to accomplish all the steps with our present system.

This example reveals the kind of probing that is necessary for a thorough analysis of each step of the process. Sometimes the answer to a "why" question will require more research. In the above example, the team could not answer the fourth "why." The team moved quickly past the surgery patient and found that the instructions were complicated and confusing.

The fishbone diagram in Figure 3-2 gives a close approximation of the team's situation. It doesn't reveal the answers, just the situation. The answers come from further exploration (brainstorming, surveys, observation, quantitative, or qualitative data gathering) after the situation is clearly understood.

The fishbone diagram is developed to make the process clearer. Once the situation is understood by all, each of the team members is able to con-

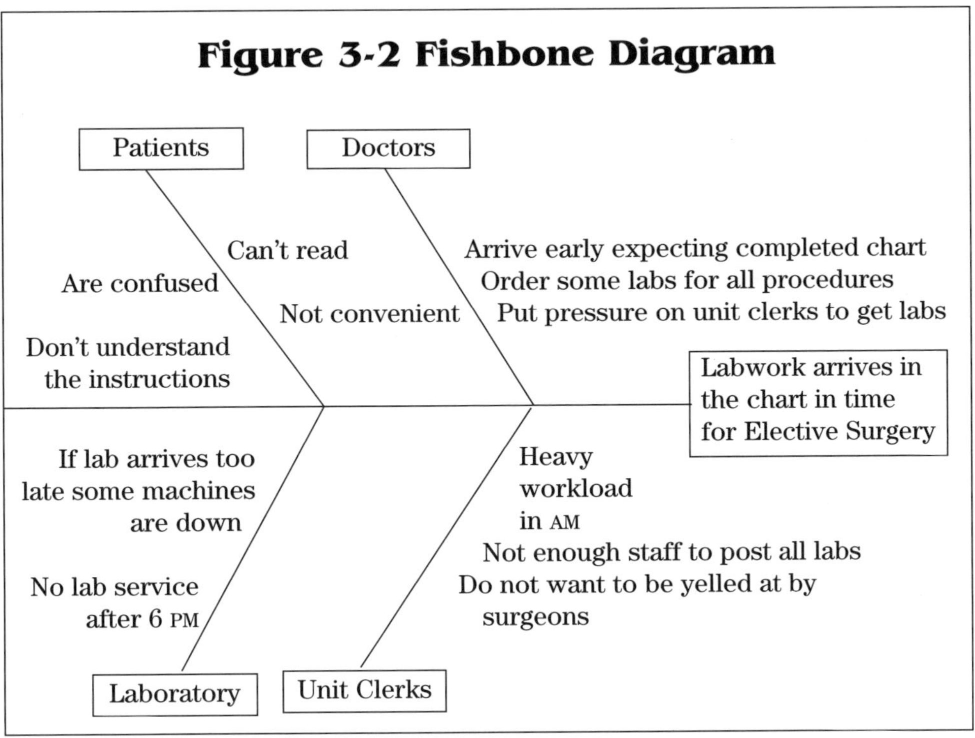

tribute to improving the process, thus improving performance and outcome.

The recommendations: The patient suggests that they get a simple oral explanation to help clarify the written instructions. The surgeon reveals that the lab work can be done several days before the scheduled operation to allow more flexibility. The unit secretaries agree to come to work an hour early to dedicate themselves to posting the lab slips. The nurses suggest that some of the labs are unnecessary for a given set of procedures. The surgeon agrees, and the number of labs is reduced. The lab agrees to use the backup machine to do any late arriving labs to avoid waiting for the primary machine in the morning.

Once the issues are clearly defined by the key players in the process, it is far easier to solve the problem. In his book *Guide to Quality Control* Ishikawa mentions the following about the fishbone diagram:

1. The creation process itself is educational. It facilitates discussion and people learn from each other.
2. It helps a group focus on the issue at hand, reducing complaints and irrelevant discussion.
3. It results in an active search for the cause.
4. Data often must be created.

5. It demonstrates the workers' level of understanding. The more complex the diagram, the more sophisticated the workers are about the process.
6. It can be used for any problem.

Top-Down Flow Chart

The top-down flow chart is perhaps the easiest way to graphically illustrate a process. The major steps are listed across the top of the page and the subcomponents are listed below. This type of diagram serves two main purposes. First, it lists the steps in chronological order. Second, it establishes, from the start, a clear dependency of one step of the process on another.

The top-down flow chart can be produced without the aid of brainstorming, but it is more effective when used in conjunction with one of these techniques. Each of the steps should be numbered as you see in Figure 3-3 for ease of tracking and reference at a later date.

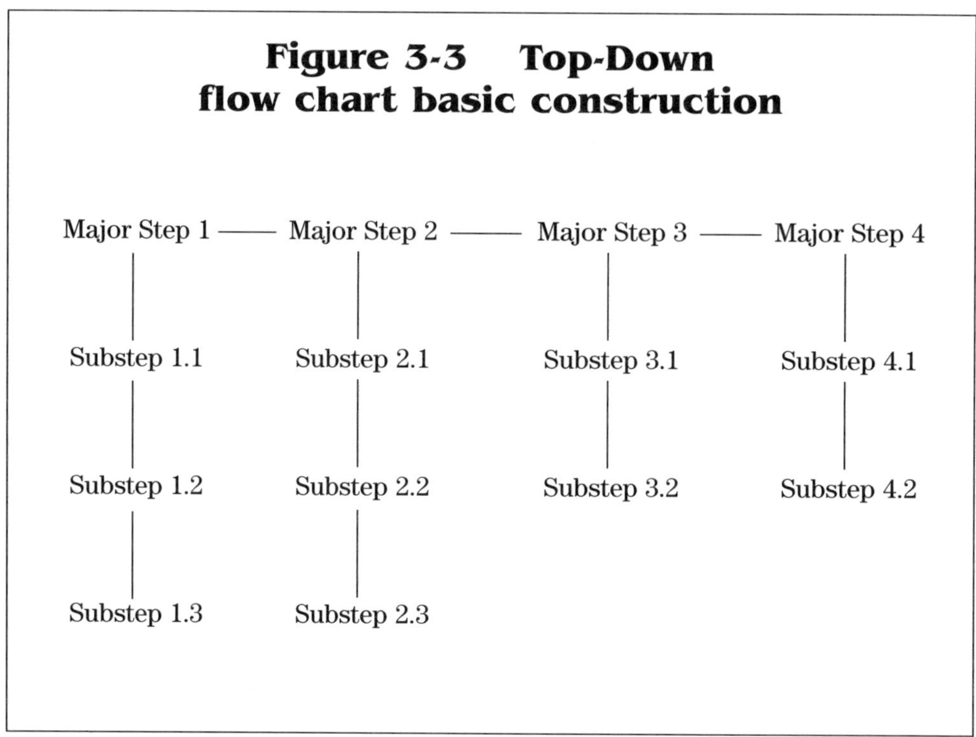

Figure 3-3   Top-Down flow chart basic construction

Process Flow Chart

The detailed process flow chart is used to analyze the decision matrix of a process (Figure 3-4). There are standard symbols for each part of the flow chart. An oval represents the beginning and end point of the process. Always begin a flow chart by identifying the start and finish points. Action steps of the process are depicted as rectangles and flow in the order of the process. Every process has decision points, shown by a diamond. The answer determines whether the process continues to flow or not. When a decision needs to be made, the question is placed in a diamond shape and response leads to the next appropriate step. Developing a detailed flow chart is a tedious process. Many times it is unnecessary to use this technique. Consider a detailed flow chart when the group lacks understanding of a complex process.

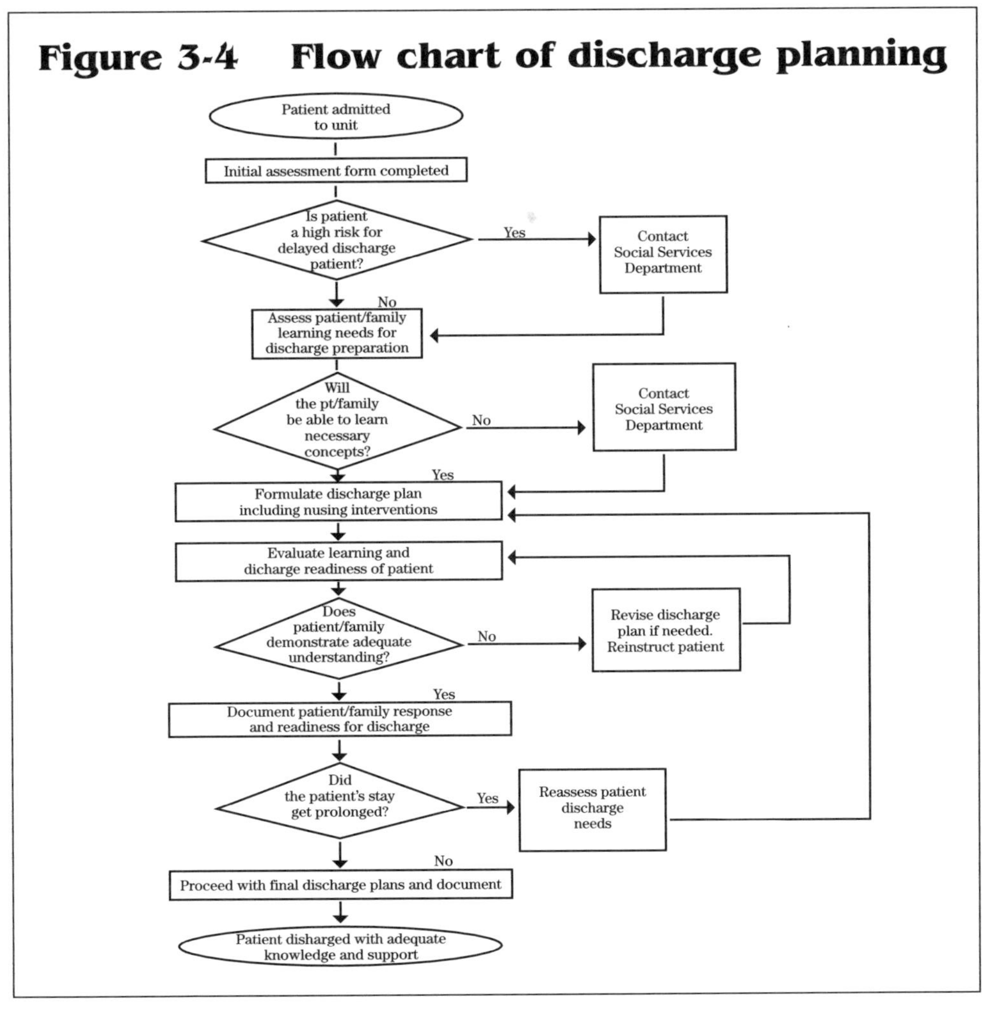

Figure 3-4   Flow chart of discharge planning

II. Team Activities

25 Cent Tour

The 25 cent tour is a very effective way to meet team members and to become familiar with other work environments. The 25 cent tour should be mandatory for all newly formed teams. It is amazing what can be learned. "I didn't know that!" or "Why do you do it that way?" are heard often along the tour.

How to conduct a 25 cent tour:

1. Schedule the tour for the second or third team meeting.
2. Make sure that all team members know they will be responsible for explaining their own area.
3. Gain permission from each area supervisor before the tour date. Be sure to emphasize that the purpose of the tour is for familiarization only, not for inspection.
4. Keep each visit sort—fifteen minutes at the most. Address issues that are relevant to the proposed project. Have fun and allow time for questions.
5. While in the area, try not to disrupt the work place.
6. After the tour, discuss impressions of each other's work place.
7. Document suggestions by group members for improving subsequent tours.

Data Collection

The data collection phase of the improvement project should be planned and managed carefully. Care must be taken to collect meaningful data. Try to ask useful questions in surveys, count the appropriate entries in chart review, and always conduct your research in a non-threatening, professional manner.

Time studies are particularly threatening to employees. They may be suspicious of management's motives and may feel that leaders are anticipating mistakes. We advise that the employees' permission to conduct the study be received first. Explain its purpose, and emphasize that the process is being examined not the people. Ask for their input and incorporate it in the data collection. Consulting the employees will prevent friction and ill will towards Performance Improvement efforts.

There are three basic ways to collect data: surveys, focus groups, and check sheets. We will discuss each one as an option the team may use to gather needed data.

Survey Techniques

Surveys are a common way to collect opinions and demographic data. A few points for conducting a useful survey are:

- List objectives for the survey and determine what data would be meaningful. Only ask questions which are directly related to the survey.
- Based on the list of objections design the survey questions so that they are easy to read and understand and will provide the desired data. Conduct a pilot study among a few people beforehand to help refine and clarify the questionnaire.
- What kind of data is being collected? For qualitative data, ask open-ended questions. Instead of asking questions, "Do you like the food?," ask "What do you like about the food?" The first question elicits only a "yes" or "no" response, while the second version yields a more helpful answer. Sorting through this data requires sound content analysis methodology and many hours. A Likert scale (one to five rating) is the standard method for measuring the subject's level of agreement to a given statement. Multiple choice surveys are convenient for the investigators, but they should be avoided because they tend to direct the subject's answers, and valuable data can be lost.
- If needed, ask for demographic data at the end of the survey. Respondents are often unresponsive to a survey if the first block of questions asks age, sex, etc.
- Always start with a cover letter containing a brief explanation of the survey and its purpose. Thank the participants ahead of time and tell them that their input is vital to the Performance Improvement process. If the information can remain anonymous, state this in the letter. People are more apt to give honest responses if they do not have to identify themselves.
- Most importantly, have the CEO sign the letter. This lends a great deal of power and credibility to the survey.
- Expect a staggered response to the survey. Send out reminder cards to participants who do not respond in one week, and then send another reminder card after two weeks. On each card, remind them of the survey's importance to the organization and thank them for participating. Again, include the CEO's signature on the cards. Be sure to include a postage free or pre-stamped envelope for the return of the survey.

Focus Groups

Focus groups are group interviews that are time-limited, open-ended, and are intended to gather responses from a small group of people regarding a specific topic. Groups typically include six to eight people and may last up to two hours. While focus groups have been used in the past for many types of research, they are also becoming an effective way to gather information from patients regarding health care services, programs, and provider-consumer relationships. Focus groups can also be comprised of hospital staff to elicit responses on new programs, outcomes and process improvements.

Beaudin and Pelletier provide five steps for executing focus groups in health care settings.

Step 1. What to question?
The questions to be asked need to be clear from the onset. This can include problem identification with service delivery or product use, or feedback regarding a service or product during planning stages or before implementation. Clear questions will help focus the interview and provide a framework for the questions.

Step 2. Who is the target population?
The unit of analysis, or the individuals who make up the focus group, needs to be determined based on the questions and the topic to be explored. This may include patients (consumers), employees, physician groups, hospital board members, or employees of customer organizations.

Step 3. How and where is the group organized and facilitated?
A written protocol should be developed for the focus group. The time length of the group, location, and questions to be asked should all be standardized. There should be two or three predetermined questions to guide group discussions. In addition to a group facilitator who promotes response and discussion, a transcriber is needed to take accurate notes. Tape recordings or videotaping can be used, but these devices often inhibit people from talking freely. Notes are crucial because they contain needed data.

Step 4. What should be done with the data?
The focus group discussions are transcribed and the content is examined for any themes or recurrent concepts. The data can be analyzed by a variety of methods, such as individual raters, tabulation of word or phrase frequency, and summary of conversation content. One drawback of data analysis is that it can be very time consuming.

Step 5. Did they really say that? What does it mean?

Findings should be communicated in written form and through oral presentations to the various work force members that could benefit from the focus group data. The patient's point of view, presented in his or her own words, can be a powerful message. Both positive and negative data can pinpoint processes needing improvement, outcomes that did not meet expectations, and systems of care that may need to be redesigned to better benefit the patient.

Check Sheet

A check sheet, or score sheet, rewards the frequency of an occurrence during selected observations. The check sheet is employed in most statistical analysis and is easy to understand and use. The team first must decide what specific data needs to be gathered and the time period during which the data will be collected. A check sheet form is then constructed, with clear directions and definitions for its use. It is a good idea to pilot the check sheet to verify that it is actually gathering all the data needed. After the pilot testing, the individuals who will be collecting data need to be trained in using the form. Every time the event occurs, a check is entered in the appropriate category. At the end of the data collection period, the forms are gathered, and each row and column is tallied for analysis. Check sheets can be used with direct observation for events, chart review, or any type of data when the frequency of the occurrence needs to be maintained. Remember, the data will only reveal how often an event occurred, and not why it did or did not happen. Data gathered by check sheets, surveys, or focus groups need to be further analyzed in order to derive appropriate conclusions. There are several simple data analysis tools which will help a team understand what the numbers imply. The principles of these tools are renewed in the next section.

III. Data Analysis

Pareto Chart

The Pareto chart is based on the 80/20 rule which states that a few of the causes (20 percent) account for most of the problems (80 percent). The Pareto chart is extremely helpful to the Performance Improvement team because it graphically represents this principle in an easily understood way.

The chart itself (Figure 3-5) is a series of bars that represent, in descending frequency, the occurance of a certain problem or situation. Identifying the tallest bars, which account for most of the problem, will direct improvement efforts to areas where they can be most effective.

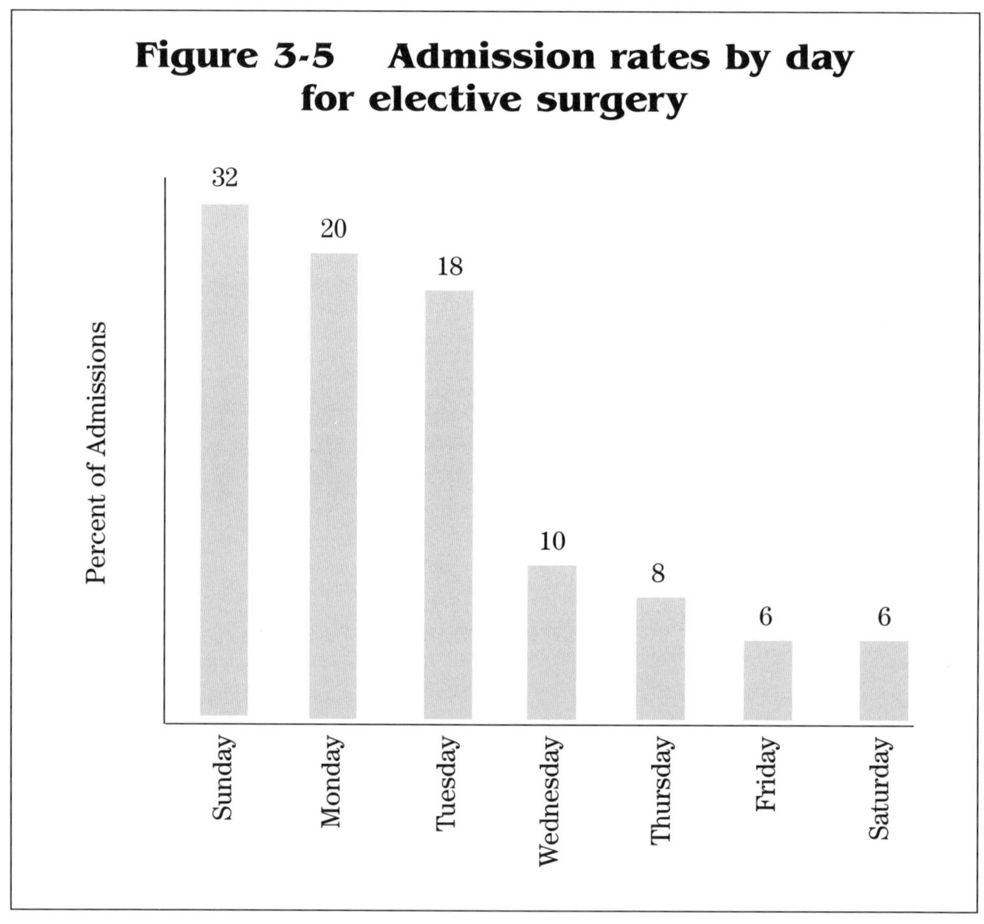

A second generation Pareto chart breaks down a selected problem even further into its own set of problems. Creating a second generation chart may be necessary when the problem is too complex to attack with a few simple steps. Pareto charts can also be useful when comparing frequency of occurrences before and after actions for improvement have been taken, in order to evaluate effectiveness.

Scatter Diagram

The scatter diagram (Figure 3-6) is used to test if two variables are related, to determine causes of process problems, and to illustrate how one variable affects a second variable.

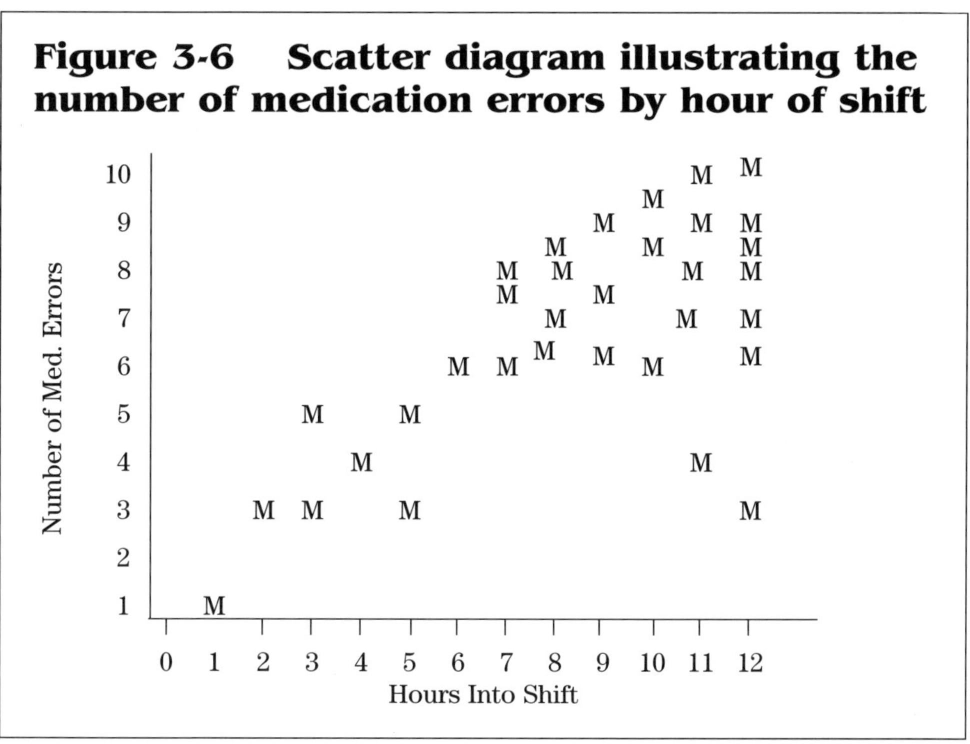

Figure 3-6   Scatter diagram illustrating the number of medication errors by hour of shift

The steps to construct a scatter diagram are:

1. Determine the variables (cause/causes or the cause/effect)
2. Obtain paired data (low reading, high reading, and several points in between).
3. Place the cause on the horizontal axis.
4. Place the effect on the vertical axis.
5. Plot the data.
6. Check for patterns. Patterns can be interpreted as positive correlations, no correlations, or negative correlations (see Figure 3-7).

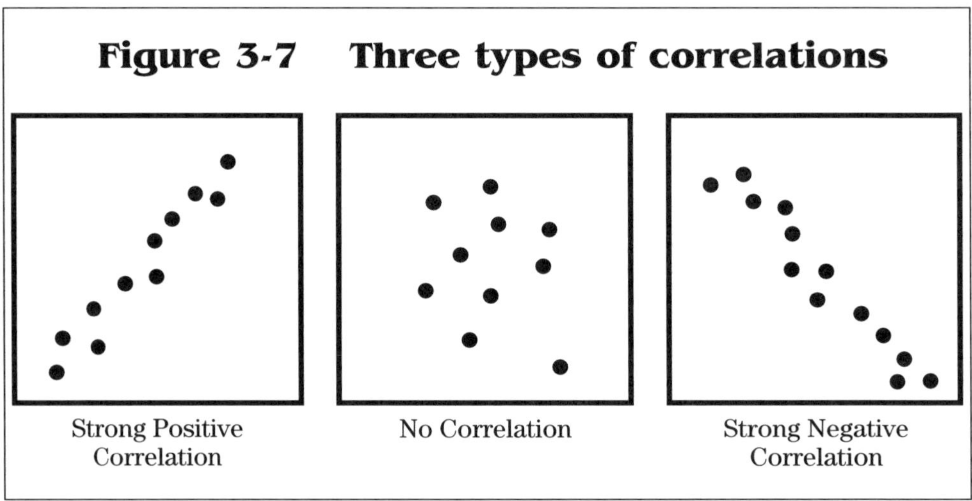

Run Chart

A run chart is designed to follow trends in the variables being observed. In nursing, the standard temperature, pulse, and respiration chart is a classic example. Run charts can be useful tools for a Performance Improvement team when trying to determine if patterns or trends exist in data. Run charts can also reveal if a trend has changed after an intervention.

Control Chart

The control chart displays the expected range of variation in a stable process. A process is stable when all the data points are within the stated control limits. Many organizations use this chart to monitor steps in a process that are prone to variation and may affect the quality of a product or service. Performance Improvement teams can use control charts to determine if the process is performing in the way it was designed.

Every process has variation, which is referred to as common cause variation. Common cause variation is expected and is illustrated in a control chart by data points falling within the control limits. Special cause variation indicates that the process is not performing as designed, and that certain factors have caused the data points to fall outside the control limits. Whenever special cause variation occurs, an in-depth analysis is needed to determine what has happened to alter process outcomes.

The upper and lower control limits can be set at one, two, or three standard deviations above and below the mean. The type of process and outcome being studied will determine how many standard deviations the data will be allowed to fall between. In health care, most processes deal with human outcomes; thus, one or two standard deviations away from the mean should be an acceptable amount of variation. If data stays within the control limits, then the process is stable. When data falls outside the control limits, the process is unstable and the variation needs to be investigated.

Initially, almost all processes will be unstable until steps are taken to reduce errors and variation in the process. For example: The nurses on the oncology unit have reviewed their patient satisfaction data and discovered that many patients were complaining about the length of time between their admission to the hospital and the start of chemotherapy. Initial data analysis of the process revealed that over a one-month period, 40 patients had been admitted for chemotherapy, and the average time between admission and start of chemotherapy was 4.65 hours. Data were analyzed on a run chart, initially, to identify trends.

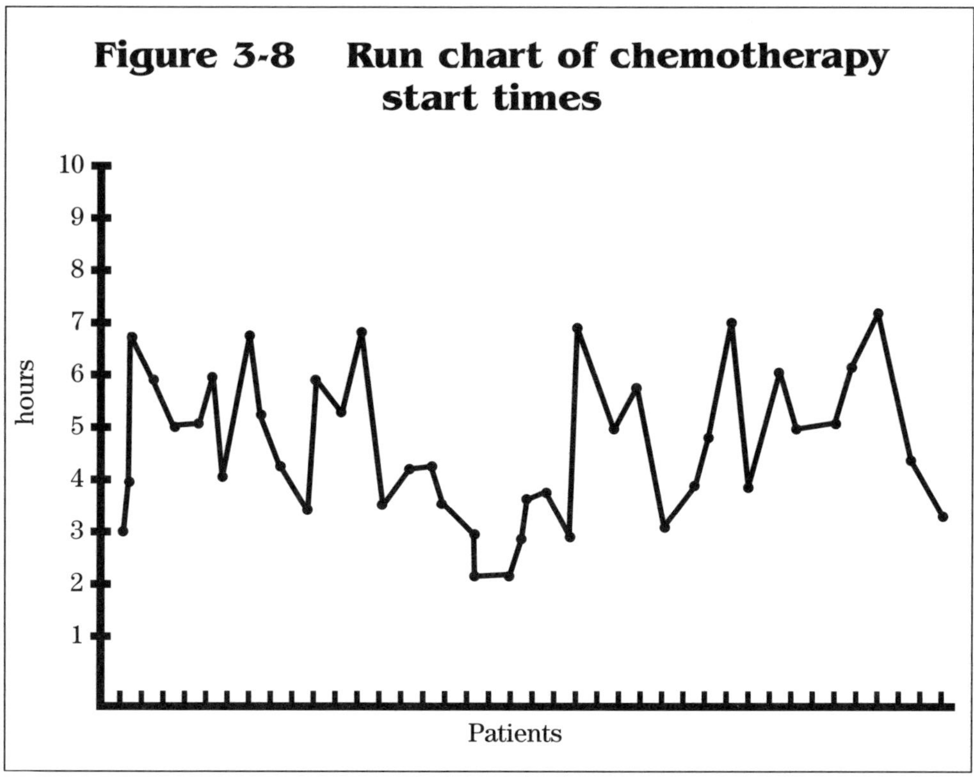

Figure 3-8   Run chart of chemotherapy start times

A Performance Improvement team was formed to examine the process. The team consisted of two oncology nurses, the unit pharmacist, a pharmacy chemotherapy technician, a unit coordinator, and an oncologist.

They reviewed the current process by constructing a process flow diagram and brainstorming for possible reasons for delaying the initiation of chemotherapy.

From the previous data, a control chart was made setting the upper and lower control limits one standard deviation above and below the mean. The chart gave the team a clear picture of how often the process was currently outside the limits or out of control. The team was able to determine appropriate actions and target their efforts for improving the process (see Figure 3-9).

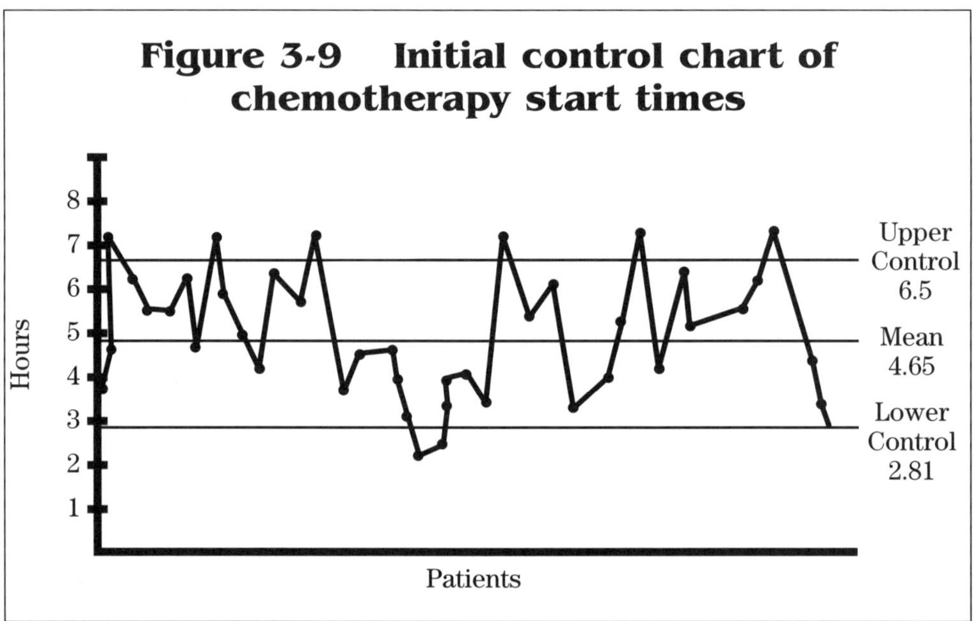

Figure 3-9   Initial control chart of chemotherapy start times

A second control chart constructed three months later revealed that all the data points now fell within the control limits; thus the suggested and implemented changes in the process had successfully decreased the time of starting chemotherapy after admission (Figure 3-10). The Performance Improvement team agreed to periodically measure the chemotherapy start times to ensure that the process remained stable.

What if, after a year or so, the control chart showed several data points outside the control limits? These occurrences would, by definition, be considered special cause variations. Special cause variations do not occur nor-

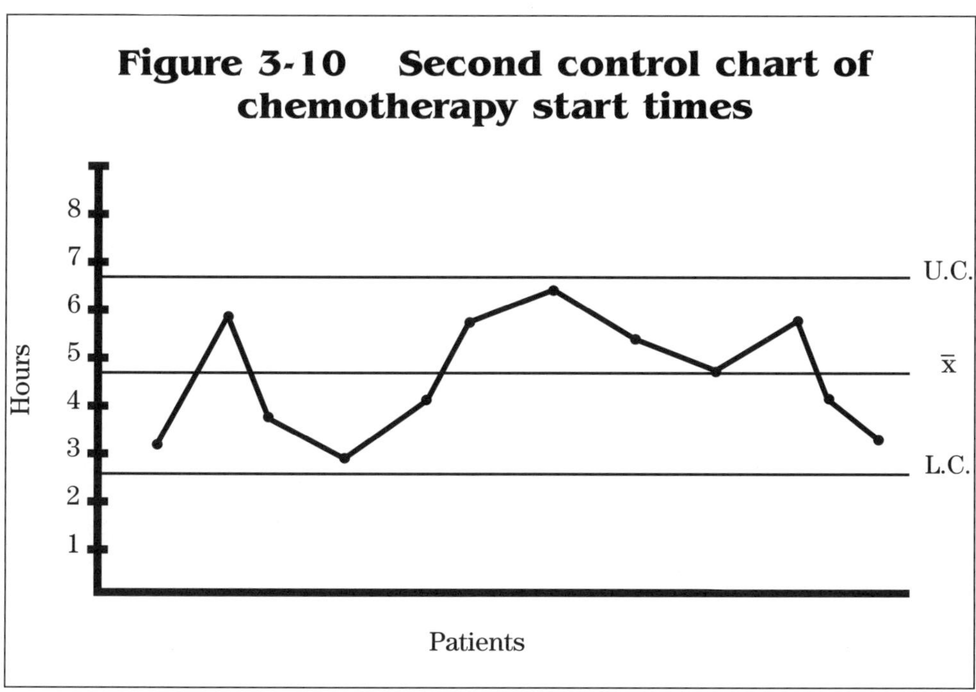

mally in a stable system and are usually caused by uncommon factors. In this case, data outside the control limits triggered a new investigation by the team to identify what changes in the process. It was discovered that a new oncologist was admitting patients to the unit. He admitted all of his patients on the same day of the week and told them all to arrive at the hospital by 8 a.m. By the time he had admitted all his patients and written chemotherapy orders, three hours had elapsed since their arrival to the unit. Upon discovering this, the team shared the information they gathered with him. The oncologist subsequently modified his admission practices to establish a more timely process.

Histogram

The histogram measures the shape of the frequency and the pattern of your data over time. Categories are prioritized in a histogram as they are in a Pareto chart. Use the histogram when interested in the shape of the distribution of a variable (Figure 3-11). A normal or "bell curve" shape suggests that the process is working as designed, while abnormal shapes suggest the process needs attention.

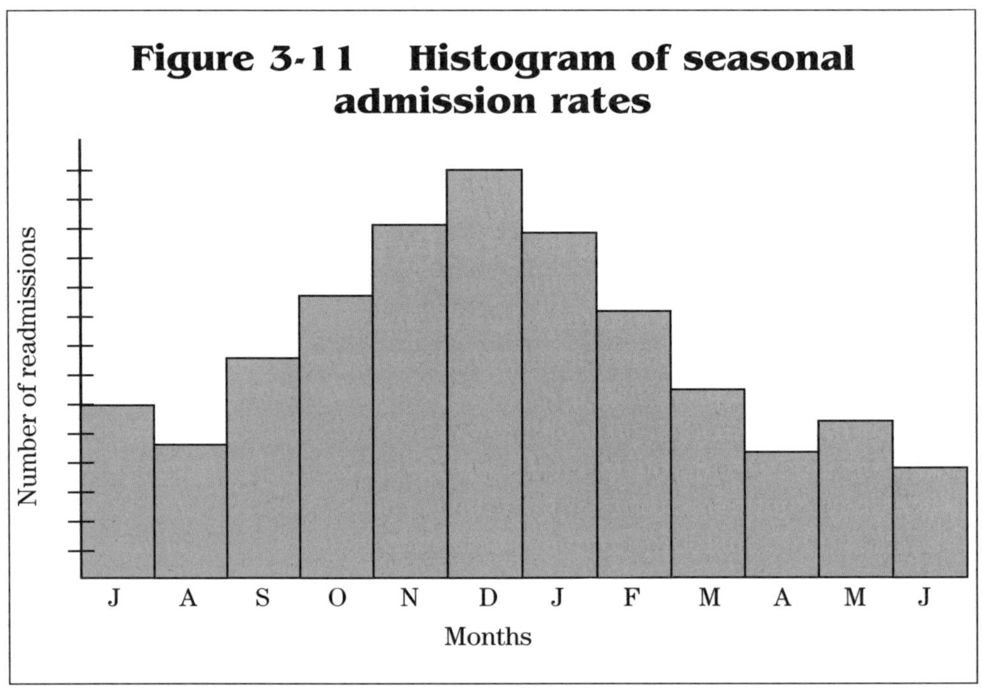

Figure 3-11   Histogram of seasonal admission rates

Action Steps Based on Facts

Once a problem has been identified and researched, the Performance Improvement team is ready to present its recommendations to the Performance Improvement council or senior leadership. The presentation of the findings and recommendations should be impressive. The elements of an effective presentation are:

I.   Introduce the Performance Improvement team by name and work location.

II.   State the problem as directed by the Performance Improvement council.

III.   Briefly describe the situation using either a simple flow sheet or a fishbone diagram.

IV.   Briefly discuss the data collection techniques and tools.

V.   Present findings using Pareto charts or other statistical tools. List major achievements accomplished by fixing obvious system problems.

VI.   List recommendations based on findings. If appropriate, show the impact of your suggestions on manpower, training, supplies, and budget.

VII.   Ask for approval from the Performance Improvement council to implement your plan.

VIII. Acknowledge team member contributions.

The audience will probably include the executive group, fellow Performance Improvement team members, the quality advisor, and invited guests. Remember to talk to the executive group. Look at them directly, make them feel important, and thus gain their respect. Keep the presentation under 30 minutes as the average adult's attention span is approximately 20 minutes.

If the presentation was effective, most of the recommendations will be well received. However, not all of the suggestions will be approved. Remember to provide the Performance Improvement council with updates, and they will be able to judge if suggestions should have been approved. Present the information in three ways:

1. Talk with them,
2. Show them slides, overheads, or presentation boards, and
3. Give them the information in writing.

When the Performance Improvement council has heard the presentation and approved the recommendations, the plan can be implemented.

Plan for Implementation

Presenting a project, in which much time and effort has been invested, to the public can be exciting. Use the following tools to help effectively implement the plan with minimum confusion.

Time Line

The time line is a series of project deadlines along a continuum. It is helpful to use the time line as an outline in developing a more detailed deployment chart (Figure 3-12).

Figure   3-12 Time line

	Aug	Sep	Oct	Nov	Dec	Jan	Feb	March	Apr
Step 1	⟶								
Step 2				⟶					
Step 3							⟶		
Step 4									⟶

Education and Training

Even the best laid plans will not work without adequate education and training. Do not forget this important step. Many good ideas have failed because the staff hasn't had adequate training. The training should be non-threatening and relevant to the task. Early in the process, establish behavioral objectives by which to teach and evaluate. Behavioral objectives state, in clearly defined terms, what can be accomplished during a given instruction period. The objective should be measurable. For example, "After completion of the class the student will be able to list four signs and symptoms of cardiac tamponade."

If the students cannot list the four signs and symptoms of cardiac tamponade, then they have not met the standard and will need to study over. Without a clear course of instruction that supports the plan, the entire project will be delayed, or dropped.

Tips on Implementation

Start Small

A good piece of advice is to "think big but start small." Employees should resist the temptation to present all their ideas at first, although they may have visualized a final grand project. Start with a small project that will be well received and successful. This project doesn't have to be a top priority, but it must have some positive impact. Save the heavy hitting projects for when the organizational climate is right. The benefits of an early success are obvious—the work force will always join a winning team.

Measure Performance Closely

Once the project is underway, measure its progress closely. Whenever a meal is served in a restaurant, the waiter or waitress will come back after a few minutes to check if there are any problems. They do this to correct errors early before patrons become frustrated with an incorrectly cooked meal or poor service. Evaluate project milestones and talk with the team members to assess their level of understanding and involvement. Don't interfere, rather, be a supportive influence.

Strongly encourage both good and bad comments. Feedback from team members is crucial because they may have suggestions to improve the process that were not considered in the planning stage. They may also have questions about the new system that can be answered, thus preventing errors and misunderstandings before they happen.

Make any necessary minor or major alterations. Mistakes are made even with thorough planning. The key is to admit the mistake, correct it, and move on. The employees will think more highly of a leader who is able to admit the mistake, rather than blame the system or an individual.

Documentation and Tracking

Process Improvement Tracking Format

After the process has been clearly defined, improved, and set into motion, a format to document the success is needed. Documentation is a necessary task; however, paperwork should be kept to a minimum because it takes time and money away from providing quality service. Completing the blanks of the form "seals the deal" like a contract. Processes, responsibilities, and dependencies become clear once in writing.

The process improvement tracking (PIT) format should replace the policy and procedure (P&P) manual. The PIT format implies that the document is temporary. One month or one year later, an employee may suggest a better idea, and a new improvement method may be implemented.

A busy staff nurse will not have the time to convert all P&Ps to the process improvement tracking format. It is suggested that the upper two levels of management be responsible for this task. Think of this document as a strategic planning tool for those who have leadership roles in the organization.

This format works well with word processing programs or with database applications. Anyone versed in basic database programming can manage to fill in the blanks of the form. A database program can produce reports based on revision dates, departments, or any other information entered in the file.

To organize the management of the PIT, a process number will be identified for each document. This number will be linked to facility vision statements, department identification codes, year groupings, issue numbers, and the number of associated agreements. An example of a Process Improvement Tracking template is as follows:

PROCESS IMPROVEMENT TRACKING
(NAME OF HOSPITAL)

(TITLE)

DATE:
PROCESS NUMBER:
PRIMARY RESPONSIBILITY:
SECONDARY RESPONSIBILITY:

IMPACT CHART:

Supplier
Supplier
Supplier   ⇨   Nursing Action   ⇨   Service to Patient
Supplier
Supplier

AGREEMENT SECTION:

OBJECTIVE:
EQUIPMENT:
PROCEDURE/FLOW CHART:

| Major Step 1 | ⇨ | Major Step 2 | ⇨ | Major Step 3 | ⇨ | Major Step 4 |
| Substeps . . . | | Substeps . . . | | Substeps . . . | | Substeps . . . |

TOLERABLE VARIATION IN PROCESS:
NEXT REVISION DATE:
TEAM MEMBERS:
AUTHOR:
AGREEMENTS:

Explanation of Process Improvement Tracking template:

**BUTTERFIELD MEMORIAL HOSPITAL
COLD SPRING, NY**

TITLE (of process)

DATE: (date of preparation of document)
PROCESS NUMBER: 4.101.9001.1,2,3

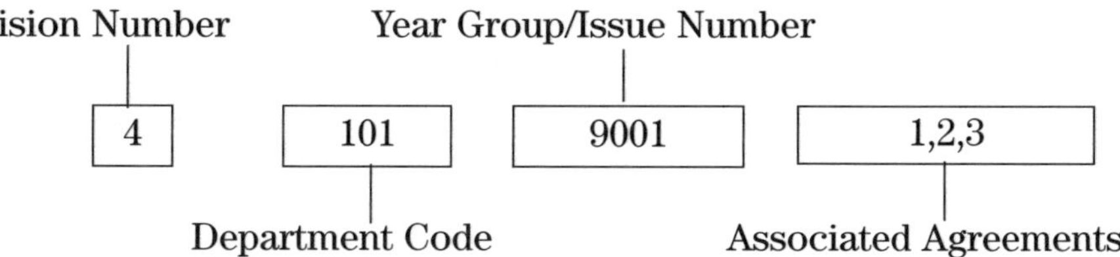

PRIMARY RESPONSIBILITY: (Who or which department is in charge)
SECONDARY RESPONSIBILITY: (in the absence of the department in charge)
IMPACT CHART:

Supplier
Supplier
Supplier   ⇨   Nursing action   ⇨   Service to patient
Supplier
Supplier

AGREEMENT SECTION:

OBJECTIVE: (a brief statement of the expected outcome of the process)
EQUIPMENT: (Specific materials, preferred brand names if necessary)
PROCEDURE/FLOW CHART: (top-down flow chart of nursing action)

Major Step 1   ⇨   Major Step 2   ⇨   Major Step 3   ⇨   Major Step 4
Substeps . . .   Substeps . . .   Substeps . . .   Substeps . . .

TOLERABLE VARIATION IN PROCESS: (Acceptable flexibility within process)
NEXT REVISION DATE: (next time to review process)
TEAM MEMBERS: (employees responsible for this draft)
AUTHOR: (primary author of this document)
AGREEMENTS: (name and number of all associated agreements)

Sample of a Process Improvement Tracking template:

**BUTTERFIELD MEMORIAL HOSPITAL
COLD SPRING, NY**

**TRIAGE AND CARE OF "SPRAINED ANKLE"
IN EMERGENCY ROOM**

DATE: 6 July 90
PROCESS NUMBER: 4.101.9001.1,2,3
PRIMARY RESPONSIBILITY: Charge Nurse, Emergency Room
SECONDARY RESPONSIBILITY: Staff Nurse, Emergency Room
IMPACT CHART:

Supplier		**Nursing Action**		**Service**
Physician on duty				
Radiology service	⇨	Nursing triage of sprained ankle	⇨	Correct and timely care of sprained ankle
Orthopaedic service				

AGREEMENT SECTION:

OBJECTIVE: The head nurse will assess, triage, and start care for all patients presented to the emergency room with a sprained ankle within ten minutes.
EQUIPMENT: Compression bandage, ice, wheelchair, crutches

PROCEDURE/FLOW CHART:

1. Neuro-Vascular System		2. Immediate Care		3. Diagnostic Tests		4. Physician Intervention
1.1 Check affected extremity for sensitivity to light touch, if intact, go to step 2.1. If not, notify physician immediately.	⇨	2.1 Apply ice, elevate and immobilize. 2.2 Provide crutches or wheelchair.	⇨	3.1 X-ray request for ankle series per physician's approval. 3.2 X-ray exam within fifteen minutes of presentation to Radiology Dept.	⇨	4.1 Obtain patient's X-ray. 4.2 Place patient in exam room. 4.3 Notify physician.

TOLERABLE VARIATION (Exceptions) IN PROCESS:
1) Initial assessment time can be longer in life-threatening emergencies which require nursing services.
2) Radiology services may be delayed due to caring for a more urgent patient.
3) If only one sprained ankle, a crutch is acceptable, but a wheelchair is preferred.
NEXT REVISION DATE: 6 Oct 90
TEAM MEMBERS:
Jane Smith, Head Nurse, ER
Fred Jones, Staff Nurse, ER
Mary Contrary, M.D., Chief Emergency Service
Fred Flinstbone, M.D., Director, Orthopaedic Service
Jennifer Gamma, M.D., Director, Radiology Service
AUTHOR: Nancy Supervisorioro, Ambulatory Nursing Supervisor
ASSOCIATED AGREEMENTS(S):
ERMD/4.101.002
ORTHO/4.101.124
RAD/4.101.208

BUTTERFIELD MEMORIAL HOSPITAL
COLD SPRING, NY

TRIAGE AND CARE OF "SPRAINED ANKLE"
IN EMERGENCY ROOM
AGREEMENT BETWEEN ER PHYSICIAN AND ER NURSE

DATE: 6 July 90
PROCESS NUMBER: 4.101
AGREEMENT NUMBER: 4.101.002

IMPACT CHART:

Supplier		**Nursing Action**		**Service**
Physician on duty	⇨	Nursing triage of sprained ankle	⇨	Correct and timely treatment of sprained ankle

AGREEMENT SECTION:

OBJECTIVE: To establish a nurse-physician triage and treatment management strategy for patients presenting to the emergency room with a sprained ankle.

PROCEDURE (4.101):

1. Neuro-Vascular System		2. Immediate Care		3. Diagnostic Tests		4. Physician Intervention
1.1 Check affected extremity for sensitivity to light touch, if intact, go to step 2.1. If not, notify physician immediately.	⇨	2.1 Apply ice, elevate and immobilize. 2.2 Provide crutches or wheelchair.	⇨	3.1 X-ray request for ankle series per physician's approval. 3.2 X-ray exam within fifteen minutes of presentation to Radiology Dept.	⇨	4.1 Obtain patient's X-ray. 4.2 Place patient in exam room. 4.3 Notify physician.

TOLERABLE VARIATION IN PROCESS:
1) The physician reserves the right not to accept the nurse's assessment of the patient's condition.
2) In the event of urgent patient care situations, the physician may not be able to order a radiology exam within 10 minutes.

SPECIAL INSTRUCTIONS:
The ER physician agrees to allow the triage nurse to assess patients presenting to the emergency room with a sprained ankle per process number 4.101.
The nurse, as an extended care provider, will demonstrate knowledge and skill of the appropriate assessment of a sprained ankle to the director of emergency services or a designee before this certification is granted.

NEXT REVISION: 6 July 91
AUTHOR: Martha Washington, R.N.

REPRESENTATIVE SIGNATURES:

NURSING SERVICE ____

EMERGENCY MEDICINE ____

**BUTTERFIELD MEMORIAL HOSPITAL
COLD SPRING, NY**

**TRIAGE AND CARE OF "SPRAINED ANKLE"
IN EMERGENCY ROOM
AGREEMENT BETWEEN RADIOLOGY AND
EMERGENCY SERVICES**

DATE: 6 July 90
PROCESS NUMBER: 4.101
AGREEMENT NUMBER: 4.101.208

IMPACT CHART:

Supplier		**Nursing Action**		**Service**
Radiologist and X-ray technician	⇨	Nursing triage and treatment of sprained ankle	⇨	Correct and timely radiography of sprained ankle

AGREEMENT SECTION:

OBJECTIVE: To establish an Emergency Room–Radiology Department treatment management strategy for patients presenting to the emergency room with a sprained ankle.

PROCEDURE (4.038):

1. Present Patients to Radiology		2. Accept and Review X-ray Request		3. Perform X-ray Exam		4. Discharge Patient
1.1 Acknowledge presence of patient. 1.2 Give waiting time. 1.3 Send ER escort back if not needed.	⇨	2.1 Check order for completeness. 2.2 Check diagnosis with requested exam. 2.3 Call ER if any questions—document reasons for call.	⇨	3.1 X-ray request for ankle series per physician's approval. 3.2 X-ray exam within fifteen minutes of presentation to Radiology Dept.	⇨	4.1 Obtain patient's X-ray. 4.2 Place patient in exam room. 4.3 Notify physician.

TOLERABLE VARIATION IN PROCESS:
1) The physician reserves the right not to accept the nurse's assessment of the patient's condition.

2) In the event of urgent patient care situations, the physician may not be able to order a radiology exam within 10 minutes.

SPECIAL INSTRUCTIONS:
The ER physician agrees to allow the triage nurse to assess patients presenting to the emergency room with a sprained ankle per process number 4.101.
The nurse will demonstrate knowledge and skill of the appropriate assessment of a sprained ankle to the director of emergency services or a designee before this privilege is granted.

NEXT REVISION: 6 July 91
AUTHOR: Martha Washington, R.N.

REPRESENTATIVE SIGNATURES:

NURSING SERVICE ____

EMERGENCY MEDICINE ____

4

Outcome and Data Management

Health care organizations collect volumes of data, typically in many different departments. Risk Management collects data on incidents, falls, and medication variations. The Utilization Review department tracks patients' length of stays and readmission rates per DRG. The Epidemiology staff measures nosocomial infection rates, needlesticks, and TB exposures. These are just a few sources of data within the hospital. What do we do with all this data? After all, data are only numbers. Performance Improvement programs need to define what data are important to the organization. PI teams will determine what data are necessary to measure process outcomes and performance. Thus, the overall purpose or goals of the performance effort will define which data are needed and why. This is called data management, and is defined as "the process of establishing data needs, retrieving and analyzing data and linking data to desired outcomes." (T.P. Williams)

Data are a key element of any Performance Improvement process. In the JCAHO "Cycle for Improving Performance," data are crucial in each of the four steps. In the first step, **design,** reliable valid data are required before any plans or objectives can be drawn. **Measurement** is the second step, and it is defined as the process by which data are collected. The goal of measurement is to provide data that objectively describes how a process is functioning. Transforming data into information is the third step, **assessment**. Assessing data means translating data into information in order to draw conclusions about performance and identifying any variations in outcomes. Analysis of the data can lead to assessment and conclusions. The last step is **improvement**. Any process redesign effort is going to be based on previous data and conclusions. The improvement efforts success will be evaluated by comparing the previous data to the present data.

Measuring Outcomes

There are two ways of measuring outcomes. Measurement of selected important processes in nursing are calculated on a continuous basis. For example, patient satisfaction surveys provide monthly or quarterly feedback. Medication variances, adverse side effects, and nosocomial infections are all outcomes that are also continually being measured. When an issue has been identified for a Performance Improvement team to review, measurement on the priority issue or outcome is done. This second type of measurement is time limited and is a more intensive assessment of the outcome and performance.

Determining which outcomes are going to be measured depends on the priorities set by the organization. A traditional method of deciding what outcomes to measure is by identifying:

- High risk processes—such as certain procedures that are a risk to the patient. These must be performed correctly every time.
- High volume processes—such as discharge planning.
- High problem or problem prone processes—such as fall prevention programs.
- High cost processes—such as open heart surgery and organ transplants.

Another way to determine which processes may be chosen for improvement efforts is to identify a weak process that is causing problems for the organization. For example, the process of getting patients to the physical therapy department was complicated involving many steps and various communication channels (see Figure 4-1). Often patients arrived late for their physical therapy appointment, resulting in shorter treatment times or no treatment at all.

This process breakdown was costly for the organization in several ways. First, loss of treatments meant loss of revenue. Second, if physical therapists were waiting on patients to arrive, they were idle and nonproductive. Patients and physicians were also not happy with the current process because missed treatments often resulted in lengthening patients' recovery and length of stay. This process became a priority for a Performance Improvement team to review and redesign to achieve better outcomes. Data regarding the number of late patients were gathered before and after improvement efforts to evaluate if the outcomes had improved. See Figure 4-2.

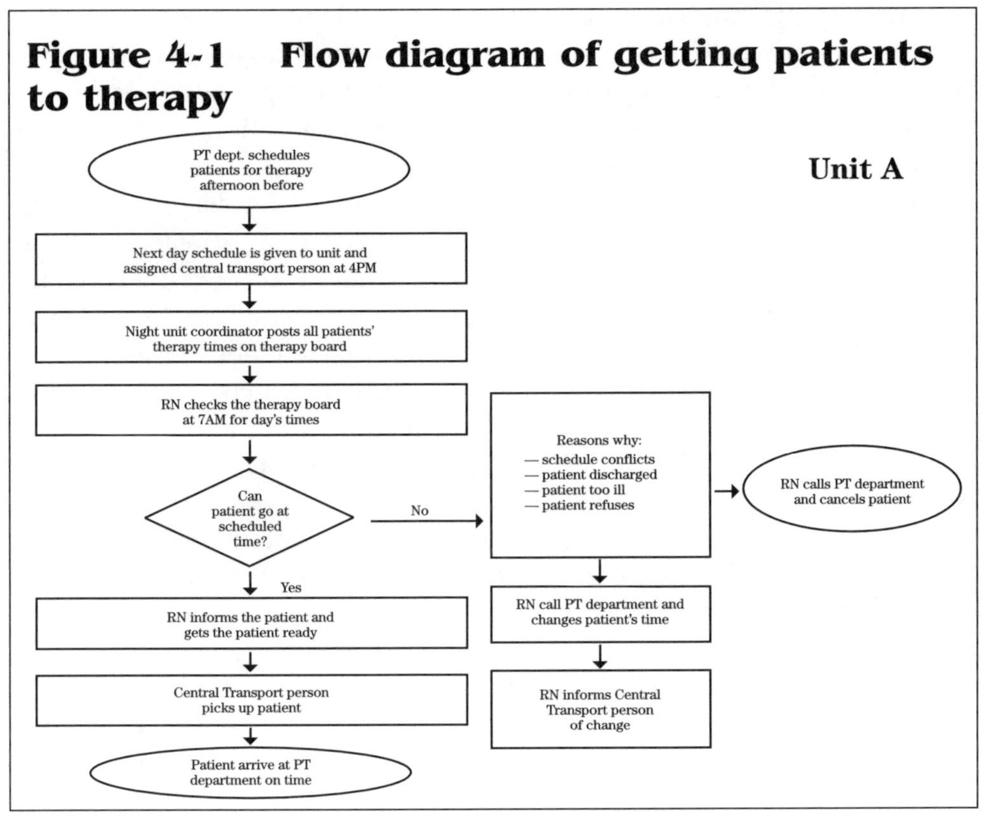

Figure 4-1 Flow diagram of getting patients to therapy

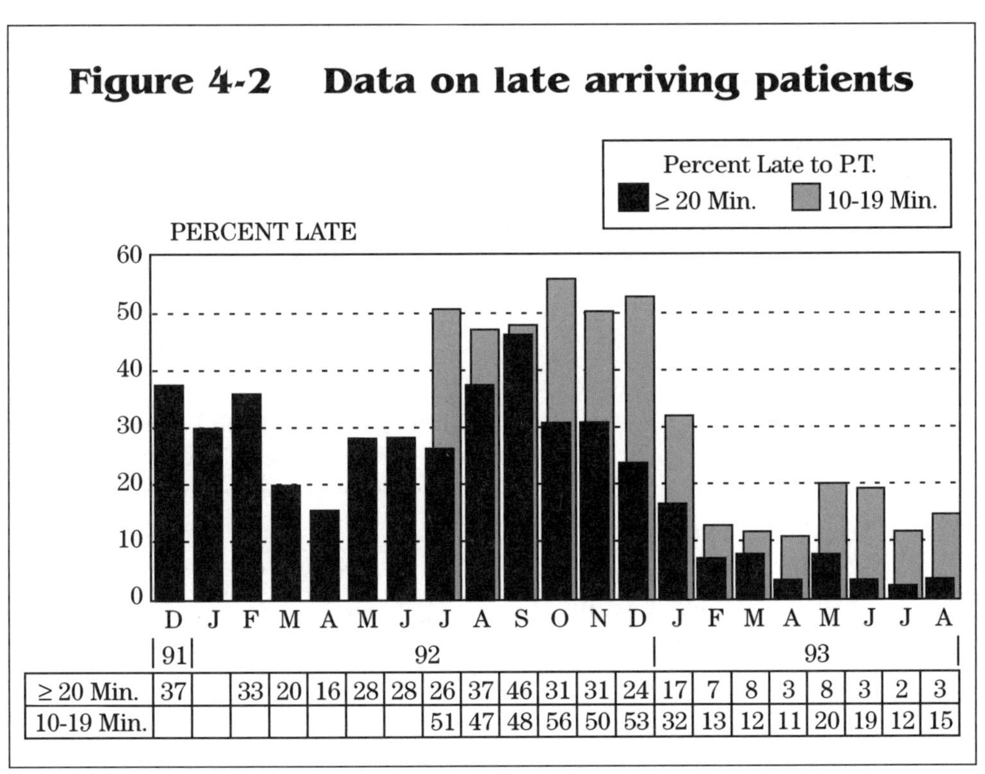

Figure 4-2 Data on late arriving patients

	D	J	F	M	A	M	J	J	A	S	O	N	D	J	F	M	A	M	J	J	A
	91					92											93				
≥ 20 Min.	37		33	20	16	28	28	26	37	46	31	31	24	17	7	8	3	8	3	2	3
10-19 Min.								51	47	48	56	50	53	32	13	12	11	20	19	12	15

The organization may want to look at a stable process that is adequate but needs improvement as a guide for further efforts. Many times these outcomes are identified through staff or patient satisfaction surveys. Improving the process could improve the level of service satisfaction. An area which always receives some negative comments from patients is dietary. What typically happens is the patient is ready and able to eat, but his or her hunger does not coincide with the food service schedule. Most patients do not like to have to wait for the meal to be ordered, prepared, and delivered. Keeping a variety of food on the unit, which can easily be prepared and served to the patient, improves this process and the patient's satisfaction.

Selecting a process that is linked to a negative outcome is an obvious choice for measurement and improvement. Reviewing pain management data can assist in identifying current practice and areas to improve. This is also true for fall prevention programs, skin assessment protocols and IV site infection rates. Each of these processes could potentially result in negative outcomes for patients if they are not adequate or appropriate. Thus, they would become high priorities for outcome measurement and improvement efforts.

The leadership of an organization must set the priorities for improving performance. Nurses can be influential in identifying processes needing improvement because they are the ones closest to the patients and clinical outcomes. Senior leaders need to be made aware when undesired outcomes are occurring or processes are no longer effective. This will assist them in determining the focus of the organizations' PI efforts. For this communication to occur, the leadership must create an atmosphere in which staff feel permitted to acknowledge areas needing improvement without fear of any negative consequences.

Data Management Plan

No matter what process is selected or outcomes identified for measurement, a data management plan is needed. There are six key components which the PI team should review prior to gathering data. Good planning will help the team get the information needed for analysis. The six steps are as follows:

Data Management Plan

1. Define Data Needs
2. Identify Data Sources
3. Identify Performance Measures
4. Study Design
5. Data Retrieval
6. Data Analysis

Step One: Define Data Needs

This step is needed to define the topic. Specifically, what processes and outcomes need measuring. Remember, the organization is a system of departmental functions that are integrated and related to other departments. Functions are made up of many processes and yield many different outcomes. It is important to choose the outcome that most closely measures the topic of concern. For example, if one wanted to evaluate the process of discharge planning, there are many different outcomes which could be studied. Readmission rates, length of stay, discharge teaching, and home health referrals are just a few. The team must decide which outcome or outcomes are most appropriate for the topic. If a new patient discharge teaching program has been started for patients with congestive heart failure, measuring patient knowledge would be the most direct outcome of the process as opposed to readmission rates because many different factors could influence readmissions.

One should also identify if the topic is a high volume diagnosis or procedure or if the process is high risk or problem prone. Once you have decided on the topic, here are eight questions from the *National Association of Healthcare Quality: Guide to Quality Management* the team should address:

- What data will be collected?
- When will the data be collected?
- Where in the process will the data be collected?
- How long will the data be collected before initial analysis?
- Who will collect the data?
- How will the data be collected?
- How will the data be analyzed?
- What and by whom will training be conducted?

Step Two: Identify Data Sources

Don't be too hasty to go out and collect data. Once the outcomes have been selected, the team should investigate whether data are already being collected in the organization. Utilizing data that are currently being generated will be less time consuming. Typically, hospitals collect a lot of data on a variety of topics. The team should identify the most likely source of data for their study purpose. For example, it may be from patient interviews or surveys, chart reviews, observations or a combination of sources. It is important to determine if the data sources are available, and if so, are they available on a time limited basis or are the data ongoing?

If the data are not readily available, then the team must construct a data retrieval methodology of their own. Data collection must be objective and systematic. Objective means that the data must not be influenced by the person gathering the data, and systematic refers to the concept that data needs to be collected the same way by all the data collectors.

There are two phases of data collection. First, is to choose the most appropriate method and instrument to collect information on the variables being studied. Data needs to be quantifiable. In other words, one must be able to measure or count data in order to analyze the results and make comparisons. Many of the concepts to measure are subjective feelings such as pain, anxiety, and satisfaction. Tools are available to measure such subjective concepts in a quantifiable way. For example, Figure 4-3 illustrates several pain scales which can be used to have patients rate their pain levels. These scales generate a number response. These numbers can then be compared and scientifically analyzed where as adjectives or feelings cannot.

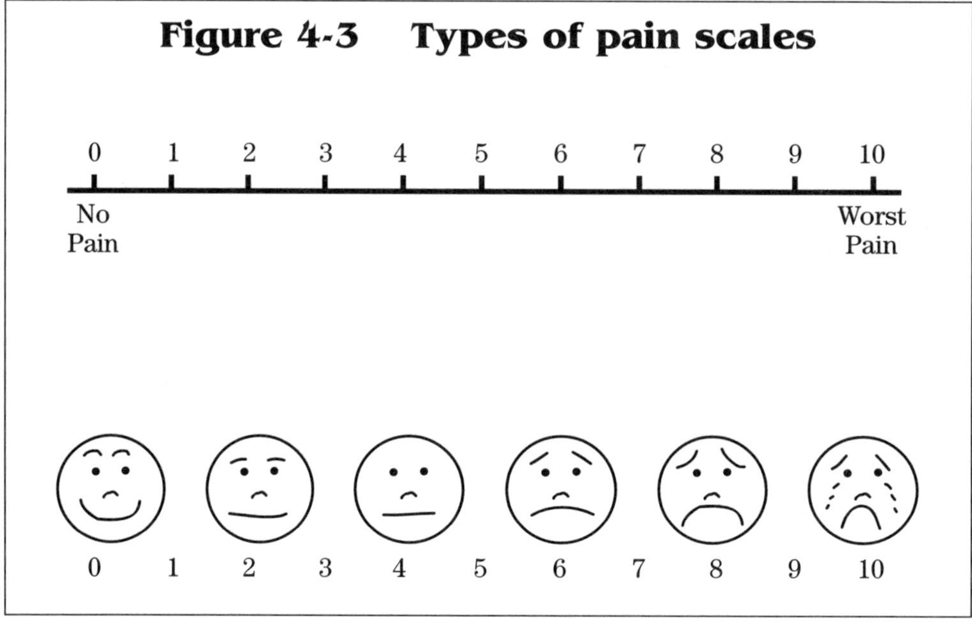

The second phase of data collection is to decide how the data collection tool will be used. Consistency is the key factor in this phase. Consistency is defined as data collected from each source in exactly the same way. For example, if the data source is a patient interview, every patient needs to be asked the same questions in the same manner. Consistency helps assure that the data are both objective, systematic, valid, and reliable.

Step Three: Identify Performance Measures

Once the topic and data source have been selected, specific performance measures need to be written. Base your performance measures on the current literature and best practice. The level of performance of the system should also reflect current standards of care and appropriate clinical guidelines. An excellent source of clinical practice guidelines is from the Agency for Healthcare Policy and Research. This is a federal agency which gathers clinical information from experts on a particular topic, such as pain management, and based on the current research, the group determines guidelines for practice and desired outcomes. These guidelines are available to everyone and are specific to certain clinical areas. At present, there are 18 different practice guidelines available.

Performance measures need to be written as objective measures. An example would be research or study questions. Here are some basic rules to follow when forming a research question:

1. Start with a simple question.
2. Ask an active question. "What is the frequency of using non-pharmacologic pain relief measures in postoperative patients?"
3. Ask a question and not a statement. A statement of fact demands no action but a question does.
4. Don't ask yes or no questions as they are not action oriented. Instead start questions with "what" or "why."
5. Don't begin questions with "should" or "could." This will typically elicit yes or no responses.

Active questions require some form of observation or measurement for an answer. One must observe something, participate, or question someone to get data on the performance measurement. An active question will provide direction for the team to answer the question in a measurable form. In addition, identify goals for your performance measures. Goals may be set using internal or external benchmarks. Goals are not thresholds, but are unique points of performance to the organization and are decided upon by the team.

Step Four: Study Design

The next step is to determine who needs to be asked the questions in order to get a measurement of performance. Some measures will require the entire patient population. Examples of this would be patient satisfaction surveys, hospital-wide nosocomial infections, and all patients readmitted within 30 days. Other performance issues may be measured by using a sample of the population. It is less time consuming to study a sample, but the researcher needs to make sure the sample adequately represents the population being studied.

One way to ensure adequate sampling is to make sure the sample is large enough. You may want to determine a percentage of the total population for your sample. Current minimum sample size is 5 percent or 30 items, whichever is greater. This rule is fine if the total population is large enough that a percentage will result in an adequate sample size. However, the smaller the frequency of the event being studied the larger the sample needs to be. Taking a small percent of the total will not provide valid, reliable data.

Step Five: Data Retrieval

A data collection plan must be developed after the sample has been chosen. This plan will identify who will collect the data, when the data will be collected, and the actual format or data collection tool. Again, look at the data sources that already exist within the organization. Available resources in terms of people and systems should be identified at the beginning of the study. Also, prior to initiating the study, the cost of doing the study must be compared to the potential gains. Cost includes time, people and other resources required.

Another important point is to decide whether the data collection will be concurrent or retrospective. Retrospective data collection means the events have already occurred. These type of data can easily be gathered through chart reviews and can be done at the convenience of the data gatherer. The problem with retrospective data is the time lapse between when events occur and when any improvements can be made. Concurrent data, on the other hand, are data retrieved while the events are actually happening. The collection period may not be the most convenient, but actions can be taken immediately to correct any problems that may be identified. Figure 4-4 illustrates a retrospective data retrieval form constructed to measure parent satisfaction with a pediatric outpatient therapy clinic. Retrieval tools need to be both reliable and valid no matter which method of retrieval is used.

Reliability refers to whether the tool will consistently measure the same way every time it is used. A tool is valid if it measures what it intends to measure. Reliability and validity are concepts nurses use everyday in their clinical practice. For example, there are many clinical tasks performed daily which relate to the concept of reliability. Blood pressures and patient temperatures are repeatedly taken throughout a 24 hour period. Medical professionals trust that their data collection is reliable, and thus

Figure 4-4   Parent Satisfaction Form

THERAPY SERVICES		very poor	poor	fair	good	very good
Child's progress with	PT	1	2	3	4	5
therapy.	OT	1	2	3	4	5
	Speech	1	2	3	4	5
Home therapy	PT	1	2	3	4	5
instructions are	OT	1	2	3	4	5
helpful	Speech	1	2	3	4	5
Therapy charges are reasonable.		1	2	3	4	5
Scheduling convenient appointment times.		1	2	3	4	5
Billing statements are understandable and timely.		1	2	3	4	5
THERAPIST						
Friendliness	PT	1	2	3	4	5
	OT	1	2	3	4	5
	Speech	1	2	3	4	5
Easy to talk to.	PT	1	2	3	4	5
	OT	1	2	3	4	5
	Speech	1	2	3	4	5
Knowledgeable regarding	PT	1	2	3	4	5
my child's needs	OT	1	2	3	4	5
	Speech	1	2	3	4	5
Prompt	PT	1	2	3	4	5
	OT	1	2	3	4	5
	Speech	1	2	3	4	5
Has a positive working	PT	1	2	3	4	5
relationship with	OT	1	2	3	4	5
my child.	Speech	1	2	3	4	5
Therapist's communication with other therapists outside of facility	PT	1	2	3	4	5
i.e., teachers,	OT	1	2	3	4	5
physicians.	Speech	1	2	3	4	5
FACILITY						
Cleanliness		1	2	3	4	5
Safe environment for my child		1	2	3	4	5
Appropriate equipment		1	2	3	4	5
Location		1	2	3	4	5

Additional comments:

consistent, because clinical judgements are made about patients based on the results. Validity in clinical practice refers to the instruments used to collect information. Medical professionals need to feel confident that the sphygmomanometer is accurate in its measurement. If they are, then these are **valid** measuring tools.

Data collected to measure performance must also be reliable and valid. Many tested tools already exist in the research literature. These tools have been tested and proven to be valid and reliable. If the researcher has created his or her own data retrieval tool, then the tool may need to be pilot tested with a small sample to determine that it is reliable, valid, and truly measures the intended process.

Step Six: Data Analysis

After data are collected, information needs to be analyzed to determine if outcomes are sufficient or still need improvement. Compare current data with past performance or with former goals. The team needs to critically analyze the information before deciding on appropriate actions and responses. Also, look at what actions or improvement efforts have been tried in the past. Do they need to be changed to fit what the current data reveals? If outcomes are not being met, then the team needs to identify reasons why. Use the techniques of brainstorming, cause-and-effect diagrams, and process flow to aid in this process. These team techniques can also be used very effectively in analyzing data and identifying appropriate improvement actions.

Data are key elements of any Performance Improvement process. Understanding outcome and data management principles is vital in the making of a successful transition to Performance Improvement. Existing outcomes and data can illustrate why a change to PI is needed. Decisions for any changes need to be made based on facts and facts are supported by data. Data can assist the staff in understanding why a transition to PI is needed. Continuous measurement of outcomes can demonstrate positive effects of PI This important stage of Performance Improvement development is dependent on data management.

5

Nursing Transition to Performance Improvement

Change, especially behavioral change, is difficult. Every health care organization today is undergoing some type of change. The days of doing business "like we always have" are over if organizations want to keep up with the industry and survive the twenty-first century. Nurses have witnessed many changes in the past 10 years. For example, the acuity of patients in hospitals has increased, and nursing activities that once belonged strictly in the intensive care unit, like telemetry monitoring and certain cardiac drugs, are now practiced routinely on general medical surgical units. Patient care delivery models have gone from "primary nursing" to "patient focused teams." Such teams include non-licensed employees providing aspects of patient care which add to the overall responsibility of the professional nurse. Many hospitals have downsized and restructured departments requiring nurses to do more tasks such as phlebotomy, respiratory therapy treatments, and the transportation of patients. Some of these changes have benefitted nurses and some of them have added to their work load. All of the changes have been stressful, to some degree, because the act of changing one's behavior can create anxiety. Just like people, organizations and programs must change in order to grow.

Transitioning your traditional nursing QA program into an organization-wide Performance Improvement process will also require change. Nurses will become members of Performance Improvement tems that are made up of many other departments and professionals examining entire processes of care, not just nursing's role. Transitioning thinking from department to systems is an important change to make in order to measure overall outcomes. The benefits of using a PI program will soon outweigh the burdens of change as employees will recognize that this approach will result in higher quality and true improvements. While change is part of everyday culture, understanding some of the general concepts of change can assist in making the transition smoother for everyone.

General Concepts of Change

For organizational change to take place, there must be:

1. Discomfort, Tension, or Unhappiness with the Status Quo

Like anything else, there needs to be a certain level of discomfort and wanting to change the situation before any action takes place. Discomfort will motivate people to improve the situation. Closely examine the way work is done, the way others perform and finally, the way the customers (patients) feel about the service. Doing this will raise issues to motivate improvements.

One word of caution about the "status quo." Status quo may very well be the biggest problem to overcome. Some nurses will complain about how things are done and how they are treated. However, these are typically the same people that rebel against any changes and will say, "This is how we have always done it." Remember when making the transformation to Performance Improvement to start with a PI project that may not be a priority, but one that has an excellent chance to succeed. This will show everyone the benefits of PI and help to silence the complainers.

2. A Source of Knowledge and Expertise (Preferably, an Outsider)

Recognizing the need for help is an important virtue for everyone to learn. In the case of organizational redesign, it is extremely important. A high priced consultant who gets you motivated then leaves is not the answer. Try finding a statistician to help with the numbers. If the organization is big enough in both employees and budgets, hire a consultant with PI experience and the willingness to establish a long-term relationship with the organization. Remember, organizations will need at least three to four years to get on the right track; therefore, one session with a consultant will not suffice.

3. Education and Training for Everyone at All Levels of Responsibility

One way to minimize the discomfort with change is to make sure everyone involved knows what the changes are. Every employee will need to be thoroughly and continually educated in the basic principles of Performance Improvement. Doing this will not only educate, but motivate the work force around the central theme of PI. It will clearly demonstrate the top leadership's commitment and its willingness to invest in its employees.

The educational needs will differ among employees. The executive level will need training on creating a vision statement, for instance. Team techniques and data analysis tools may be the focus of education and training for other levels. Understanding both the concepts and application of PI tools is vital for a smooth transition.

PI education is an ongoing process. As knowledge of processes, improvement strategies, and customer expectations grow, the program will internally change. Education and training programs need to be revised to match the stage of the PI effort. An example of one management group's organization-wide education plan is as follows:

Phase 1: Introduce initial training for leaders in PI concepts and the leadership skills necessary to implement the improvement initiative, and change the organization's culture.

Phase 2: Provide education for the organization, as a whole, in the improvement initiative goals and in basic improvement concepts and tools.

Phase 3: Provide training for designated team facilitators in improvement concepts and tools, and in teamwork issues.

Phase 4: As teams are formed, offer just-in-time training in improvement tools for team members and in leadership issues for team leaders.

4. A Critical Mass of Support and Belief within the Work Force

"Here comes another change." "Something **else** we have to do." These are comments staff members may have. There will always be a few negative people, but don't let them influence the rest. Recruit them into PI activities which will make them believers in the program. Ask them for feedback on what processes they would like to see improved and elicit their assistance on PI teams. Being an active participant in change gives a sense of control, belonging, and importance. PI becomes part of the work culture and not just some new program staff are being told they have to do. Act as a model for change by being confident and positive about what is planned with a PI transition. Communication is a key factor here. Make sure everyone knows why the PI effort is important and what goals are to be accomplished. Make sure everyone knows what role he or she plays in PI. Lastly, make sure goals, activities, and achievements are regularly communicated to all levels of staff through appropriate channels. Staying informed means staying involved.

5. Adequate Resources to Get the Job Done

Performance Improvement, like any new program, requires adequate resources up front in order to be successfully implemented. These resources typically mean people and time both of which can be scarce and need to be used wisely. One way to ensure that resources are used for the greatest benefit is to set priorities for improvement activities. Focus your efforts on areas that are important to the organization. Improved outcomes, improved staff and patient satisfaction, and cost savings are all compatible goals which can be achieved through a comprehensive PI process.

Employees need to be given the time to be educated in PI and to participate in Performance Improvement activities. Without management's approval, this cannot happen. Also, PI activities can not be expected to be done in addition to regular work commitments or on employee's own time. If leadership values their PI program, then time and the necessary people must be allocated for the needed activity.

6. Leadership

Organization-wide improvement must be supported and guided by top executives. The leaders of the organization need to be persistent and determined if the transition to PI will be successful. This transition can be a slow process and one that takes commitment from all involved. It is a "continuous" improvement effort that will be revised and changed to fit the growing needs of the organization. This can be frustrating for staff because many want a one-time explanation.

Nursing leaders will play a vital role in the success of the PI program. Some suggestions for effective leadership during the transition period are:

- Leaders must communicate to their staff how improvement efforts relate to the organization's overall vision, mission, and strategic plan. This especially needs to be done in ways so that employees understand the effects on their individual roles and responsibilities.
- Leaders must demonstrate their commitment to improvements. An example of this commitment will be allowing resources for PI activities.
- Leaders must view improvement as an ongoing, integrated process and not a series of separate projects.
- Leaders need to be seen in the work place to both demonstrate their involvement in the improvement effort and show interest in staff input as an information source.
- Leaders should support PI teams by serving as a team facilitator and giving teams guidance and assistance as they proceed through their improvement project.

All of these elements will initiate the transition to a PI program. It will take some time for the transition to be completed. Periodically, the organization should reflect on the progress and identify what stage of development has been reached. This will also assist the leaders or change agents in staying focused on the goals that have been set and what tasks remain to be done. There are several stages of development in a PI process.

Stages of Performance Improvement Development

Stage 1. Shared Vision and Values Articulated through a Mission Statement

It is imperative that the commitment for a Performance Improvement effort come from the top. Without the support of top management, the PI philosophy will fail. Input from all levels within the organization is necessary to create a workable vision, but the final vision statement should come from the CEO. Once this vision is articulated, the rest of the organization must follow its tenets in every action they take. Therefore, the mission and vision as it relates to PI must be communicated clearly to the staff. This also includes informing employees of the basic priorities for improvement efforts and how priorities were set. Channels of effective communication need to be established and utilized. These will vary among organizations but could include newsletters, staff meetings, management meetings with departments and face-to-face communication with the staff. Understanding the reasons for adopting a PI process organization-wide, will help employees recognize how activities impact their own department and work area.

Stage 2. Customer Focused Culture

The customer is the epicenter of the PI organization. In health care, this may be a departure from traditional thought processes. Patients are the primary customer and their needs and expectations should be the central focus of an organization. However, health care professionals also need to determine all other "customers," both inside and outside the organization, that are served. Some of these other customers may include family members, community members, vendors, physicians, other nurses and practitioners, and administrators, to name a few. Input from these different customers must be considered when setting priorities for improvement efforts.

Stage 3. Continuous Performance Improvement Philosophy

Performance Improvement is a continuous cycle of designing, measuring, assessing and improving processes and outcomes. It is different from past quality programs which typically were time-limited and department-focused. An organization-wide PI plan will define the program's methodology and structure. Improvement activities need to be coordinated in order to eliminate duplication of efforts and to standardize the approach taken. The culture within the organization must be such that employees feel free to identify areas needing improvements and feel ownership of their PI teams. Remember, this type of cultural shift will be slow, but it must take place.

Stage 4. Education and Training throughout the Organization

The cost of quality may seem unrealistic. But PI takes time and effort—that costs an organization. The initial cost of teaching and training will be money well spent. But it doesn't stop there. Education must be continuous so that as new and innovative concepts are developed, staff can stay current in their practice. At every level within the organization, the worker, manager, and executive will have to be trained and made familiar with this new management philosophy. When planning the PI education the following questions must be asked:

- Who will provide the education?
- What topics will the education cover?
- Who will receive the education?
- What time frame will be appropriate for training?

Many hospitals have their own education department that can assist in planning the different stages and level of Performance Improvement education and training. Some pitfalls to avoid are failing to provide follow-up training after initial sessions, being too abstract, not giving concrete examples of PI efforts, and being too broad or trying to teach too many staff members too quickly. The organization may want to seek outside assistance in PI education, especially for the initial training of the principles and PI tools.

Stage 5. Clear Definition of Everyone's Role and Responsibilities

Performance Improvement is everyone's responsibility. Individual roles may be different, but everyone needs to know about the PI program and how it ties into the mission of the organization. Each person needs to know how their role fits into the overall scheme. Staff should be challenged to use their expertise and encouraged to participate in PI activities. Certainly, their efforts and achievements need to be recognized and valued. For PI to be successful, it must become part of the organization's everyday routine and not be viewed as just another "quality program."

6

Essential Elements for a Successful PI Program

Performance Improvement programs need to be organization-wide, everyone's responsibility, and embraced by a corporate culture of continuing improvement. It is up to the executives and management staff to lead this transition and set this process into motion. PI programs cannot be successful if only done by management. Employees, at all levels, must understand the principles of PI and know how it effects their work place. No matter which department nurses work in, or in what capacity, they need to understand PI principles. Nurses must become "systems thinkers" and recognize how their performance impacts overall functions and process.

An informal survey of nurse managers, cited many common reasons why nursing staff have been reluctant in the past to participate in Performance Improvement activities. Common reasons given are:

- Lack of knowledge
- Resistant to change
- Overwhelmed
- Not enough time
- Too much paperwork
- No management support
- Fear of criticism, punishment, and rejection
- Not invited to participate
- No results or benefit seen
- No rewards

There are three essential elements for a successful nursing PI program. These are **education, involvement,** and **recognition**. A cause-and-effect diagram illustrates how each of these factors can help to overcome these common barriers to staff participation.

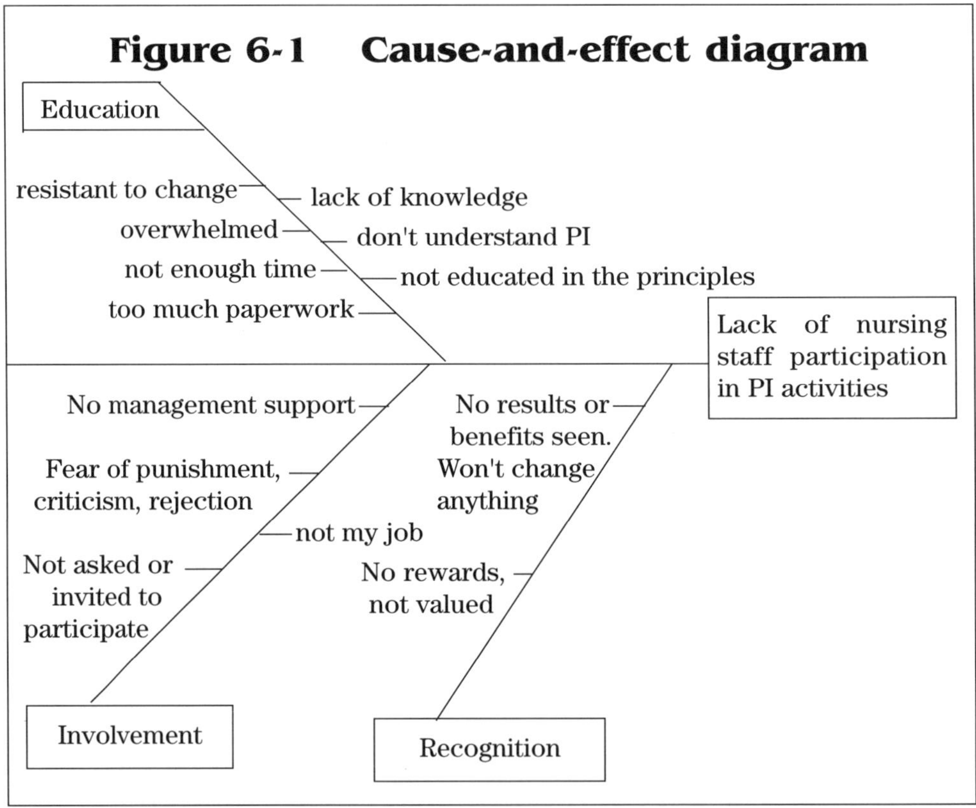

Lack of staff participation is a frequent complaint of nurse managers. Let's discuss in detail each of these reasons or excuses. Even though they are listed in separate categories, all of these reasons can be the result of the lack of education, lack of involvement, and lack of recognition. A combination of all three is needed to motivate nurses and get them involved in the PI process.

Education

Both managers and staff recognize that a "lack of education and understanding" can lead to poor participation. No one wants to accept responsibility for something he or she knows little about. This is true for

Performance Improvement activities. Nursing staff members need to be educated in PI principles with emphasis on continuous improvement, team approaches, and data management before they can be expected to participate. Education and training should be ongoing in order to address the various educational needs of the staff and the changes within your PI program. Make the training relate specifically to the organization's mission which should emphasize that PI is part of job responsibility and not just another new program. Share concrete examples of how addressing system issues and process improvements within the organization can bring changes that will result in improved performance and outcomes.

Nurses must know how a PI team functions within the organization. This includes understanding the different team roles and responsibilities. Some staff nurses may never have served on a team before, so reviewing what is expected of each team role will help them individually determine what role is best for them. Not everyone can be an effective leader, but he or she may be a very valuable team member. Knowing the different roles and responsibilities of team membership will allow staff members to succeed in the correct role for them. Training of team members on the team techniques used for problem solving is also important. Learning techniques such as brainstorming, cause-and-effect diagrams, and process flow charts will enable staff to analyze issues and identify root causes. Data analysis tools such as histograms and control charts are not skills that staff members are familiar with. Teaching staff these skills will assist them in data analysis and making appropriate decisions regarding how processes are functioning.

Methods for teaching this information can include traditional inservices and organization-wide conferences focusing on any of these PI topics. The teaching structure should fit with the underlying purpose of the education. For example, intense teaching of PI tools and techniques to prospective PI team members will need a different format than teaching the entire organization the PI process and principles. Utilizing an organization newsletter to highlight PI team successes or different aspects of the organization's PI program is an effective way to educate a large majority of employees in an easy, continuous format. Every new employee's orientation should include an overview of the organization's Performance Improvement process, model of PI and it's relationship to the mission statement and goals. This will ensure new staff members understand the PI process and the philosophy of continuous improvement.

Chapter Five states that education and training are the key for a successful transition to any change. One would expect then, that education regarding performance improvement would eliminate "resistant to change" as a factor in not participating in PI activities. Perhaps, too, the feeling of being "overwhelmed" would be lessened if staff understood the changes from QA to Performance Improvement. The PI process of team work can give staff some control over a changing environment by involving them in decision making. Educational programs on systems thinking and understanding of the processes within the organization are prerequisite before nurses can be expected to function in a PI environment. Nurses have become so isolated in their own environments that they don't realize how performance of all departments can influence overall outcomes. Nurses must possess the skills and knowledge needed to work well in multidisciplinary team settings. Training programs in communication skills, small group interaction dynamics, and delegation skills can help new team members function successfully. In addition, some nurses, especially new graduates, may benefit from programs on critical thinking skills including applying statistical principles.

In the past, QA programs were typically viewed as extra work by staff. Their arguments for not wanting to participate were "not enough time" and "too much paperwork." The arguments had merit, as QA programs tended to generate volumes of data which required a lot of staff time to collect. Then, if data were never analyzed or used, staff viewed the activity as extra paper work without any true purpose. There were also many QA meetings held only because of a requirement instead of meeting for a purpose. This was also viewed by staff nurses as an inefficient use of their time.

When PI teams meet, the purpose and intent of the group should be clearly known by the members. The team facilitator or leader should keep the team focused on the improvement issue so time is well spent. Identify data that already exists within the organization so any additional data collection is done when absolutely necessary. All data gathered should be used in analyzing process stability or identifying root causes of issues for process improvement. When PI teams are seen as adding value to the organization, the time and effort spent will not be viewed by staff as "extra work," but instead, as a necessary part of their ongoing responsibility.

The excuse of "not enough time" is very real in today's health care environment. Nurses have added responsibilities and tasks to complete. Staff members must manage their time well and prioritize their activities. PI activities must be a valid use of the staff's time. Hopefully, once nurses have learned the purposes of PI and the benefit their participation will bring, it will help them to realize this is time well spent.

Involvement

"Lack of management support" is seen as a barrier to staff wanting to participate in Performance Improvement. This could mean one of two things.

First, managers might not want staff performing PI activities because they view it as solely their responsibility. This could be true if a manager is insecure in his or her position and fears the loss of authority. But not including staff in PI processes can lead to a program with great ideas, but little actual practice. Remember, it is the staff nurses who perform many of the steps in patient care processes. If performance and outcomes are to be improved, staff members need to help identify viable solutions. The second meaning of the lack of management support comes from past nursing unit-based QA committees. Often, the entire responsibility of quality assurance was given to a select group of staff nurses. The manager did not take an active role, which gave the impression of not supporting the program. Typically, manager input was only given if the quality report was late or if data didn't indicate their department was "perfect." In this case the involvement of the manager was that of reprimanding the committee and certainly not a supportive role for staff. If the PI program has the support from management, then staff not only feel involved, but are also empowered to make decisions and become process owners.

Understanding how PI fits within the organization and, specifically, everyone's roles and responsibilities will also help staff feel involved. This will eliminate the excuse of "it's not my job" when PI is plainly illustrated as an organization-wide initiative. Many clinical staff members view their job only as those direct tasks pertaining to patient care. They may feel PI is an administrative program and not clinical. Assist these nurses in identifying areas of clinical practice and patient outcomes they would like to improve. Select one issue for improvement and have them utilize the PI process. This will show the nurses that PI activities can have a clinical focus and can also improve patient care. Relating the PI process directly to patient care will help these staff members realize it is part of their job.

Another way to show staff that PI is an organizational responsibility, is to have a flow chart which illustrates the organization's Performance Improvement program. Figure 6.2 shows one example of such a flow chart, but there can be other versions depending upon the organization.

It is up to the leaders of the organization to create an atmosphere where nurses feel comfortable to identify areas needing improvement. Staff must not "fear criticism, punishment, or rejection of their ideas." Since PI examines systems and processes needing improvement, there should not be any criticism of people or departments. No process performs perfectly, as there is always some process variation. PI efforts should be focused on minimizing variation of those processes that are key to the organization. When staff realize PI activities evaluate systems' performance and not individual performance, they will feel less threatened to participate. In a PI environment, staff will be more willing to share their ideas and become involved. Some nurses are more verbal than others and may not need to be

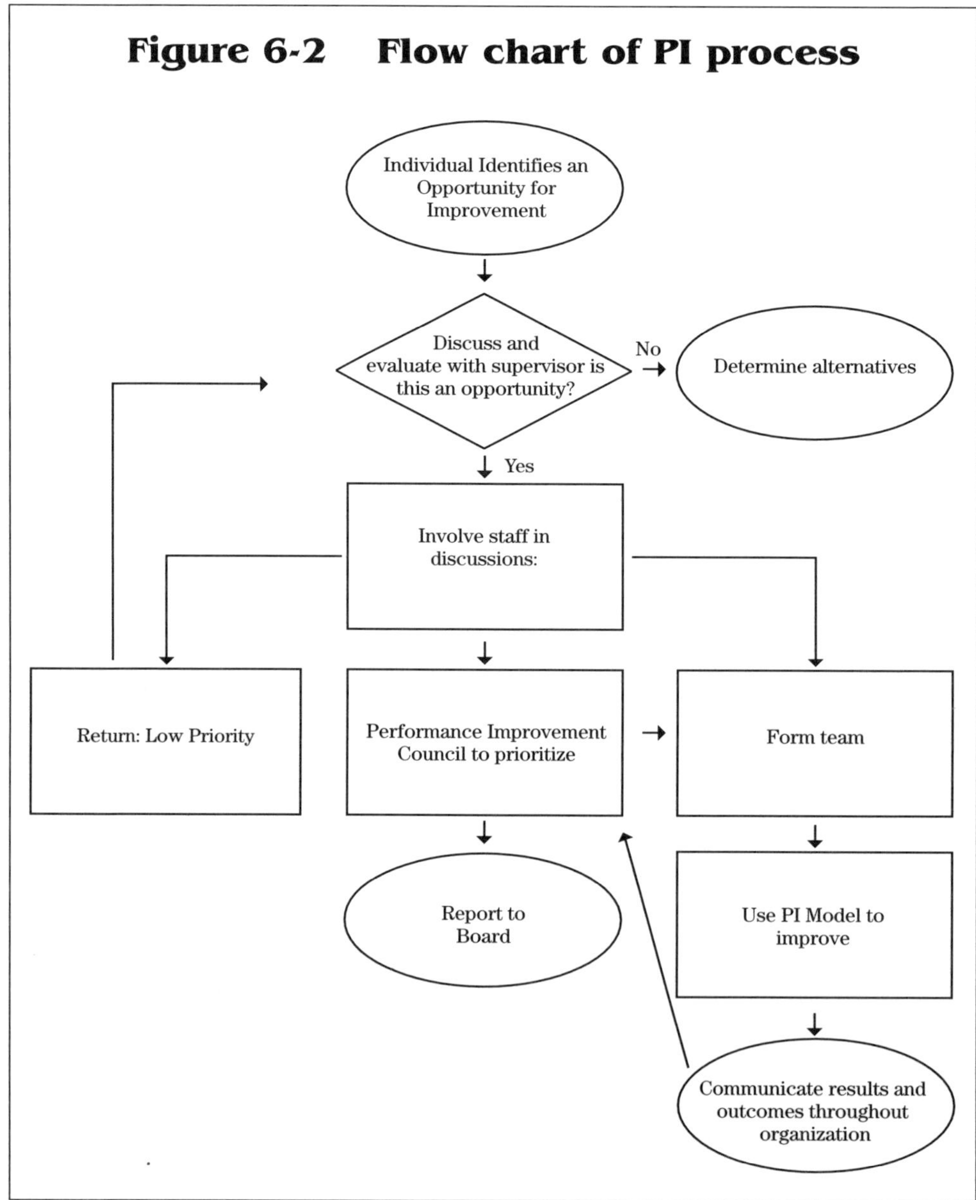

asked specifically to work on PI teams. Others may need to be invited to participate. The simple act of asking a staff member to be part of a PI team demonstrates his or her involvement is important to the PI process.

Some specific suggestions for managers to get staff nurses involved in PI activities are:

1. Take an active role in PI activities and model the principles. Know how nursing fits within the organization's Performance Improvement plan.

2. Recognize those staff nurses who possess natural leadership abilities as possible PI team leaders.
3. Identify areas of staff expertise and utilize their knowledge in reviewing processes and outcomes.
4. Redirect negativism regarding existing policies, practices and outcomes into positive, productive PI activities.

Recognition

It is human nature to want to feel valued and worthwhile. This is especially true of employees within a changing work environment. One way of feeling important to the organization is to be recognized for your efforts and hard work. Two of the reasons given for staff not wanting to participate in PI activities are "lack of rewards" and "not being valued." It is critical for a successful PI program that staff members be recognized and appreciated for their efforts. Rewards do not have to be monetary and can simply be highlighting the work of a PI team in the organization's newsletter. Other options can include having a PI team or team player honored monthly or quarterly for their achievements.

"National Quality Week" is celebrated in October. This is an ideal time to feature PI successes. One easy way to recognize everyone for their contributions is to have a poster session. Any department or PI team can construct a poster or story board of a Performance Improvement project and display it for the entire organization. Making this a contest can add to the recognition and fun. A poster session is also an excellent method of educating everyone in the organization regarding what previous performance improvements have been achieved. This may easily turn into an annual event and one that staff members look forward to as a time to learn and be recognized and appreciated.

The last reason given for staff nurses not wanting to participate was they felt there would be "no results or benefits" seen from their PI activities. With past QA activities this may have been true for several reasons. First, staff nurses were not given the authority to make decisions, so many of their recommendations were not implemented. Second, staff members were often not given all of the information needed to suggest appropriate recommendations. Thus, ideas for improvements were unrealistic because they weren't aware of all the factors involved. And last, QA activities only focused within a department and not on the entire process. Actions for improvement of process outcomes could not be identified because the process as a whole was not evaluated. With the PI process, multidisciplinary teams should be given all the facts, evaluate processes, and be able to make appropriate recommendations which will have results and benefits.

Possibly the best way to recognize staff nurses for their work on a PI team is to implement the team's decisions. When they can see their own successful results and improvements, nurses will realize the benefits and stay involved.

In order to get nurses to participate in the PI program, there needs to be education, involvement and recognition. Each element is critical in making a successful transition to an organization-wide performance improvement process. These elements are important whenever staff participation is needed. Staff nurses' participation is vital in survey preparation and the accreditation process. Thus, education, involvement, and recognition is the key for getting staff involved in these activities as well.

7

Nursing Responsibilities in Accreditation

Nurses traditionally have played a key role in preparing for accreditation surveys. The classic survey is one conducted by the Joint Commission on Accreditation of Healthcare Organizations. Nursing staff must demonstrate that Performance Improvement has become a part of a normal work day. Integrating clinical care with ongoing measurement activities is the goal. Demonstrating improvement using data must be the outcome. Measurement and data driven improvements should be system focused, collaborating with other members of the health care team.

Joint Commission standards have evolved and changed over the last several years. The most significant changes have occurred since 1992 with the agenda for change. This is when the Joint Commission began the transition to performance-based and functionally-organized standards. Standards were streamlined, condensed, and reorganized into three major sections: Patient Focused Functions, Organizational Functions, and Structures with Functions. Standards had traditionally been organized into chapters following departmental titles such as nursing, laboratory, and pharmacy. Preparation for a survey was easier and required less time when standards were departmentally based. The departmental approach did not recognize the collaboration and multi-disciplinary nature of the health care team. The new standards have led to a real-world, real-time approach to evaluating quality, performance, collaboration, and competency. Staff now have the intimidating task of reading not one, but every section in the manual.

The Start

The Joint Commission has made significant improvements in the clarity of the standards with its move to rewrite them through "Project Plain English." This alone is not enough to gain a thorough understanding of the standards themselves. To gain a better understanding, distribute the intent/preamble from each clinical section of the manual to the nursing management team as an introduction to understanding each major section. A visit from the Joint Commission does not have to create high levels of stress. A planned and collaborative process will ensure that the staff will be ready. Gaining a comfort level with the standards is the first critical step. One of the best ways to accomplish this comfort level, especially with the new emphasis on integrated standards, is to establish standards review teams (SRT) to assess how well the organization understands and is complying with the standards. Before a compliance check is initiated, however, understand the intent of the standards and know what policies and procedures support them.

The Team

Composition of the SRT is critical to successful accreditation preparation. The person selected to lead the team is the most important. These team leaders will play an essential role in coordinating the assessment of standards. It is recommended that the leaders have some background and experience with the Joint Commission survey process. The team leaders are responsible for interpreting unclear areas, leading group discussions about the standards, and stimulating discussion among team members. The team leaders become the Joint Commission process experts. Select logical process owners as team leaders. Quality directors would lead IOP, health information management director and information services would lead management of information, nursing leaders would lead care of patients, assessment, and so forth.

The standard evaluation process will require team leaders to communicate clearly the goals of the SRT. The team leader will be responsible for working throughout the organization to assess further areas the team may have identified as potentially troublesome. Nurses have traditionally been the *gatekeeper* of patient care and the coordinator of all integrated/collaborative services. Preparation for survey must focus on a demonstration of a multi-disciplinary, collaborative approach to patient care and service.

The Team Member

Team leaders cannot complete the preparation activities without good team members. Team members are the nursing and other staff who will be charged with evaluation of standard compliance and education of other staff. Nurses have played significant roles in surveys in years past and often have many members with a high level of comfort with the Joint Commission. With the new integrated standards it is necessary to review the standards across the organization to gain an understanding of how the standards apply to each and every department. A team composed of individuals representing a wide variety of departments and varying levels of management will work best to evaluate compliance with standards. Use staff that rarely are involved. Do not forget shift and weekend workers.

One of the best ways to formulate team membership is for the team leaders to develop their own list of potential candidates to serve in these important roles. Volunteers should be solicited. Do not limit team size. Spread the wealth to as many individuals as necessary to get the job done.

The Work

Evaluation of standards is the responsibility of every team member. Member assignments can be made by the team leader in advance of the first team meeting. Start the process twelve to fifteen months prior to the scheduled survey date. The goal of the SRT is to review each standard examined against nursing practice throughout the organization. The work required to evaluate a standard will vary. For example, standards in the Patient Rights section are most likely met by policies that apply to the entire organization. The team members will evaluate existing policies to assess how well they comply with the intent of the Joint Commission standard. The team member will also need to evaluate how the organizations actual practice compares with what is written in policies. Areas such as patient assessment and patient education, have traditionally been accomplished by individual nurses. The traditional departmental approach will make evaluation of these functional sections more difficult for the team member and may require discussion with other disciplines to evaluate compliance. Collaborative review will demonstrate collaborative practice.

The Meetings

Team meetings are an excellent way for team members to review and discuss their findings. A calendar for these meetings should be established that includes the dates when each team is expected to report its findings. These team members are the staff who are or soon will be the organization's Joint Commission experts. All team leaders should get together from time to time to compare notes and reduce redundancy.

Ongoing preparation is the most efficient way to achieve the very best results on a survey. Preparing staff for the survey should not be a three month period of emergency study. It is a time to help staff learn how to demonstrate areas where they have worked to improve the care. If using a mock survey tool, complete the survey three months prior to the real one. This will allow adequate time for follow-up to mock survey findings with appropriate corrections being made.

Team leaders should document all the information gathered during the work of the SRT. The team leaders should provide a report on the findings regularly. Report problem areas immediately to your Joint Commission project coordinator. There should be a in-depth discussion of standards where less than substantial compliance was found. Do not forget to review past Type I findings as those areas are certain to be scrutinized. Assignments by team leaders for corrective activities must be given to appropriate team members. Remember to review the policies that support activities leading to standard compliance.

The Organization

Your entire organization must now focus on the basics of survey preparation. Integrate the work done by the nursing SRT's with the rest of the organization. Start by preparing the first line supervisor group. Give them a good understanding of the standards, standards compliance and policies that support the standards. Use team members to provide any needed education. An effective method of providing needed education is to create a Joint Commission study review session. Here attendees will gain an understanding of the standards, know what they mean, and gain an appreciation for integration and collaboration.

Brown bag lunch meetings are an excellent forum for discussion for staff level employees. Within this framework, the group must start preparing for the actual survey. Members should be encouraged to read or at least briefly review the standards before these sessions. Key points about the standards are found in the introduction and intent section. The session leader should put into words what a Joint Commission surveyor will be looking for during a typical survey. The leader should talk about examples of implementation that are specific to your nursing unit. Use your organization-wide policy manual and relate it to your department. Staff should be able to talk about mechanisms in place in the organization to ensure access to care, appointment making systems, policies regarding denial of care, patient eligibility policies, telephone triage systems, privacy and confidentiality policies, security of medical records and medical information policies, physical security plans, and educational programs for staff on patients privacy issues. Discuss specific examples of the units' Performance Improvement activities. Review how the standards relate to nursing practice and discuss the documentation that exists to support compliance. This assists staff in updating their knowledge about policies, procedures, forms, and standards. Coordinate document review to avoid redundancy. The surveyors have not heard about what the unit has done to improve care and service. Have examples ready with data to support the improvements that have been realized.

Staff should gain a level of comfort to respond confidently to the Joint Commission surveyor questions regarding how they are personally involved in the Performance Improvement process. Each day play the 'top ten questions' game.

Top Ten questions on Improving Organizational Performance

1. Do you have a Performance Improvement program on your nursing unit?
2. How do nurses participate in PI activities?
3. Where is your model for PI?
4. Give an example of one thing that has improved as a result of the PI process?
5. Have you participated as a member of a PI team?
6. How are issues prioritized for study?
7. What system changes have occurred outside of your department that have had a positive effect on nursing care?
8. How are data collected?
9. Do you participate in data collection activities?
10. What education have you had about the PI processes?

These are the most likely questions about Performance Improvement the surveyor will ask during a survey. The Joint Commission also provides a number of helpful programs for both novice and experienced staff who need and want to increase their knowledge of standards and the survey process. Slowly your staff will begin to think, respond, and ask questions like a Joint Commission surveyor.

The Documentation

Availability of documentation is one of the critical elements to ensuring that your survey will be successful. Compile all the documents well before the actual survey. Policies that effect more than nursing areas must not be departmentally specific, but rather they should apply to the entire organization. Place policies in appropriate manuals as they relate to function. Use a master index describing what is in each manual, and index each manual separately. This manual will facilitate retrieval of the information when a surveyor asks for documentation to support compliance with a standard. Department specific policies must not conflict with either organization-wide policies or other department specific policies.

Documentation my be found in places other than the overall organization-wide policy manual, for instance, infection control manual, safety manual, or the formulary. These manuals should be placed in a location readily accessible to all staff members. These manuals should be carefully organized and reviewed before the survey. All staff members should be able to go to these manuals and find the appropriate documentation if asked to do so by the surveyor. Don't forget a user friendly index. Remember organization of these materials will pay off during the survey. The surveyor will most likely want to look over the examples of documentation to demonstrate Performance Improvement. Keep committee chairs on call during the survey to respond to any questions about minutes or committee functions.

The Mock Survey

One of the best ways to assess the readiness of an organization and its compliance with standards is to use experts for a mock survey. These experts can be from within your organization or from an outside source. Questions used during a mock survey and a listing of items to be reviewed should be developed to guide the mock survey activities. Use the "Guide to Survey" or other Joint Commission publications for sample questions. The Joint Commission publication division can help in obtaining these documents. During the mock survey, have as many members of the health care team available to role play the interview process. Such individuals may include the nurse manager, nursing supervisor, clerical supervisor, physician director, and other appropriate support staff. Listen to the questions carefully. Only provide an answer to the question being asked. It is important to emphasize from the beginning that there are no right or wrong answers. This is a chance for the staff to become comfortable with being asked questions about how to describe the provision of collaborative patient care. Use examples to support the answers. Survey participants should learn to talk about PI activities as they relate to their specific work area. Surveyors ask their questions as a patient or customer advocate. Use this knowledge to formulate your answer.

The mock survey is a time to review what to do to improve care in specific areas and to prepare answers for the Joint Commission surveyor. Support each other in front of surveyors. Don't contradict answers, even if the answer appears to be incomplete. A Joint Commission surveyor can make even the most seasoned staff member nervous. Group responses are an excellent opportunity to demonstrate collaboration. Members should be encouraged to respond to questions in the way they would respond in day-to-day communications. Don't volunteer information, always ask the surveyor to clarify misunderstood questions.

It is important to include documentation review in the mock survey process. The mock surveyor should spend some time looking for the presence of supporting documentation. Particular attention should be given to the manuals that provide guidance to staff in their unique roles. Quiz each other on department specific policies three to four weeks prior to the Joint Commission survey.

A review of the nursing unit is a critical part of the mock survey. A checklist sill assists the internal surveyor in doing a complete review. This checklist will ensure that every item is reviewed and will also serve as a guide to correction for the department nursing manager. The mock surveyor will want to inspect emergency equipment to ensure that it is secure and has been checked according to policy. Refrigerator use represents an area of potential difficulty and should be reviewed to ensure compliance with infection control policies. Fire extinguishers should have current inspections. Sharp containers should be secured. Medical records should be kept in secure places where patients do not have ready access. Any materials, like 'white boards' with patient names should be kept in places where individuals other than health care professionals cannot see them. Review the environment of care plans carefully. Place emphasis on department specific application of safety and fire emergency activities.

Questions directed to nursing staff during the mock survey should vary depending on their job responsibilities. Be ready to assemble the health care team for questioning during the real survey. Pick the physicians carefully. Find a champion. Discussions about patient assessment and care of patients will most likely take place. Any employee is fair game to be asked questions about Performance Improvement, safety, and staff rights. Use medical staff leaders to communicate with other physicians. Rehearse answering questions about collaborative care.

The Real Survey

When the Joint Commission survey team arrives, there is little more that can be done to prepare. Follow their prescribed agenda carefully. Surveyors have much to do, and not much time to do it. Always accompany the surveyors, never leave them alone. Have secretarial support available for copying or providing other tasks if the surveyor requests it.

The efforts will be rewarded by a successful survey. Keep the preparation process alive so next time preparation will be easier for the staff. Develop an internal newsletter to keep everyone informed. Continue both formal and informal team meetings to discuss standard changes and updates. Include new employees so a uniform level of understanding will be achieved across the organization.

8

Automation

When to Automate

Automation for the sake of automation is never a good idea. In general, nurses get more done and with less effort using old methods. Because it is thought to be easier. That's why staff members resist automation changes, especially when it comes to computers. Computers are highly touted for their productivity potential, communication systems, and ultimate cost savings. Situation-specific applications of this technology are not widely known or utilized.

Think about the computers in the workplace. Are they used for producing posters, invitations, and an occasional letter? Do the monitors double as a place to put the coffee maker? Do workers stare blankly into the monitor for hours at a time, tapping a few keys every now and then? In settings such as these, productivity cannot be high.

Computer technology does have a function in the workplace. The job is to find it. Here are a few guidelines to help make the right choices. Automation is right for the workplace if the answer to all of these questions is yes:

- Will the application enhance service to the customer? Or will it only benefit the organization?
  Example: Computer software that produces excellent end-of-the-month billing reports but hard to understand patient billing statements has the wrong focus.
- Will the cost of the system, applications, and training be an investment or a loss to your organization?

93

Example: Purchasing a computer system that has both too much storage space and mainframe-like software applications is too costly, is typically not easy to use, and will take nurses away from patient care.

- Does the application eliminate rework?
  Example: Software applications that integrate information to eliminate repetitive tasks such as creating bills, form letters, and periodic reports.
- Is the interface (the interaction between the computer screen and the user) intuitive? How long will it take to learn?
  Example: Poor computer interface is the single biggest drain on learning and user time. Personal computers that dominate the work environment have done little to enhance the true productivity potential of the computer. Why? Poor interface, integration, user knowledge of capabilities and time management.
  The computer should be an extension of the worker. Ideally, the computer helps do difficult tasks without workers having to learn detailed computer procedures.
- Situations and rules change all the time. Is the present computer system or application flexible enough to change without much effort?
  Example: A new computer has arrived on the nursing unit. One of the reports does not include new assessment requirements or a place to collaboratively document findings. Who will modify the program? Who has the knowledge, time, and skill? Who will provide additional training to staff? Is the computer system capable of change and expansion?
- Finally, does common sense dictate that investing resources of time and money into automation makes sense?

If you "pass the test," then there are some things to know about the alternatives. There are many types of computer hardware systems and software applications. Competition in this market place is intense, competitive, and evolving. Costs and capabilities vary widely. Understand the needs first, then match them with a compatible system.

The hardware must match the needs of the workplace exactly—shop wisely. Enlist an expert's help if you are not comfortable with these decisions. Discuss these options with information services staff.

Software applications can be grouped into several major categories. The organization should use each as a part of an integrated PI process that would ultimately serve all customers.

Database Management Systems

Database management systems (DBMS) are an excellent tool for keeping track of almost everything. Tracking a patient's address, billing, medical history, medications, and medical diagnosis are but a few examples. Most of all, DBMS helps you answer all kinds of questions: How many of the patients live in a particular area? To whom should a PAP screening letter be sent? How many patients take a certain medicine or have a certain diagnosis? Using "paper" records for these purposes would be possible, but tedious and inefficient.

When purchasing a DBMS package, remember that it will not come "ready to run." An operator must tell it what kind of information to save and how to present it. It is beyond the scope of this book to expand on DBMS design. It is recommended that interested parties find an expert in this field to explain capabilities, compatibilities, and cost. Just know what to ask for.

Statistical Packages

Statistics packages are basically the same. The companies that produce these packages would take exception to that statement, but there are only a finite number of statistical analysis variations. Most of these products are too complicated and unnecessary for PI process evaluation. PI statistical tools should be developed with a basic level of understanding and health professionals can get along fine with a basic stats software that will produce easy to understand graphs, charts, and reports.

Word Processing Applications

Word processing has proven to be a powerful feature of computers. If nothing else, it has effectively eliminated rework. Documents needing revision are easily modified and produced. Word processing packages should be implemented in every area. Purchase one that has all the latest technology. As your knowledge becomes more sophisticated, the more "complicated" features will be used and appreciated. Color printers and graphic applications make producing quality products easy.

One word of advice: Make sure to purchase the best printer possible. The word processing product is the document—make it look good off the screen. This conveys an image of high quality.

Education Source

Be careful about considering the computer as an educational source of information. Computer assisted learning is an expensive way to design a training program. Some individuals still resist computer technology. If applicable, this can be a powerful method of ongoing, self-directed, continuing education.

Affordable technology is now available. Look for computer controlled compact discs that have not only written words, but also video and audio capabilities to augment instructions. While these packages are available, experience has indicated most hospital systems do not contain the hardware necessary to run these programs, so be prepared to update the hardware systems as well.

Centralized Information

Centralized information is not a type of software but an important concept to keep in mind. The connecting of personal computers—or networking—has greatly enhanced the utility of automation in the workplace. A centralized repository of information is very important in Performance Improvement. Here are a few examples:

- Project improvement teams store their meeting agendas, complete with the latest findings and suggestions, on the mainframe network for all to view and edit.
- Inter-department communication via electronic-mail assures a fast, accurate, and secure way of distributing information.
- Customers, by way of a public access workstation, offer comments to the organization. This is an efficient way to collect market research and design customer-driven services. A terminal in the pharmacy waiting room with a very simple data-entry screen (maybe even a touch screen like those in airports and some ATM machines) and a keyboard for comments would also be a helpful way to collect information.
- Employee involvement programs are enhanced by an automated method to offer suggestions, either anonymously, or by name.
- External customers/suppliers can be directly linked by telephone or fax modem into selected portions of the organization's automation system. Suppliers can pick up orders, communicate with the users of their product, or suggest improvements in their product or service.
- Fax transmission of documents enhances both speed and efficiency

in placing and filling orders, obtaining consent, and keeping others informed about patient/organizational information.
- The "paperless" medical record is another example of centralized information technology. Quick access, security and ease of documentation highlight this growing area.

The Internet has opened doors to knowledge and communication not imagined a few years ago. Basic computer skills and equipment can link offices with the world. The following is a short list of what is available to the average user.

The World Wide Web

—Clinical Data
—Clinical Resources
—Telemedicine Resources
—Federal Government Resources
—Health Care Resources
—Professional Resources (discipline specific)
—Health Care Risk Resources
—Health Education Resources

Many of these services are free to the health care professional. Explore this option with the information management office staff.

Glossary

25 Cent Tour—A tour that introduces fellow project team members to each member's place of work.

80/20 Rule—Eighty percent of the trouble comes from 20 percent of the problems. Otherwise known as the Pareto Principle.

85/15 Rule—Eighty-five percent of the problems are due to a system error rather than an individual error.

Action List—A list assigning tasks to be accomplished by project team members for the purpose of Performance Improvement.

Agendas—A list of topics for discussion at a team meeting. This list should, ideally, be started at the end of every meeting and finalized and disseminated several days prior to the next meeting. The topics on the agenda should be prioritized and have time budgeted for them.

Automation—Occurs when a task is handled by a machine. Machines include blood pressure monitors and computers.

Bell Curve—A curve which graphically represents a "normal" distribution of data. The normal distribution traditionally includes three standard deviations from the means or 96 percent of all occurrences or measurements. All those data that fall outside the 96 percent are considered outside the system, and thus out of control.

Benchmarking—The process of comparing a product in a critical way with other competitors. To benchmark a particular service, first select which factors of the service to compare, then use these factors as the basis of the comparison. Also known as competitive benchmarking.

Brainstorming—A technique used by groups to suggest ideas in a creative, "free for all" way. A moderator simply writes down all ideas on a large sheet of paper or blackboard. The key to brainstorming is to make sure group members do not comment at all on other member's ideas. Brainstorming is used to collect ideas from a group without regard to the validity of those ideas. This approach fosters creativity among group members if the group can refrain from becoming judgmental during the brainstorming session.

Cause and Effect Diagram—See fishbone diagram.

Check Sheet—A sheet which keeps a tally of the occurrences of selected observations. Statisticians think of this as the beginning of a frequency table.

Continuous Improvement—A philosophy that strives for state-of-the-art products or service. Implies that a process and its service/outcome are never optimized.

Control Chart—A chart which displays the expected range of variation in a stable process.

Control Limits (upper and lower)—Mark the numerical boundary of variation within a process. Staying within the boundary implies a stable system.

Cost of Quality—The costs incurred due to bad quality within a given process. Concept originally defined by Dr. Joseph Juran in the 1950's.

Critical Mass—Top management must work to convince and to educate a "critical mass" of employees about PI management style. The critical mass consists of the top third of your organizational structure.

Crosby, Phillip—Developed a theory of absolute quality and zero defects. Based on the aerospace industry and focuses on quality control concepts.

Cultural Change—Refers to the paradigm shift from traditional management by results to management utilizing performance improvement process.

Customer-driven Organization—Organizations that recognize their customer/supplier relationships. In health care organizations, patients are the priority customers.

Customers—People or other organizations that use your services, i.e., patients, families, physicians, employees.

Deming, Dr. Edward W.—Some say the "founder of total quality management." Deming is a statistician who is an expert in management principles based on statistical control methodology. Deming is credited with helping Japan's post-WWII industrial base be one of the best in the world.

Detailed-flow Chart—A chart, that, through standardized symbols, illustrates in detail all the steps within a process including yes/no branches. The detailed flow chart is used to analyze the decision matrix of a process.

Employee Involvement—A phenomena of employee participation closely linked with "empowering of the work force." Employee involvement is a key factor in a successful PI organization.

Empowerment—In an organizational setting, it is the assignment of ownership of a process to an employee. The three main ingredients of work force empowerment are: 1. participatory in nature, 2. influence without authority, 3. rewards and performance systems.

Evaluation—Evaluation of a system or process should be done with quantitative data. Evaluation of an employee should be more subjective and provide feedback on how they can improve.

Facilitator—A role in a PI team. Assists the team leader and facilitates group processes and productivity. A gatekeeper.

Fishbone Diagram—A graph which demonstrates the cause and effect for a given outcome. The effect is the desired outcome and the cause(s) are the "spines." The common variables are manpower, money, materials, and methods. Use the fishbone diagram during situation analysis.

Fitness for Use- - Juran's central theme for quality improvement. The customer defines/dictates what is "fit for using."

Function—A goal-directed, interrelated series of processes.

Histogram—A bar chart that displays the shape and frequency of selected data over time.

Ishikawa, Kaoru—The author of the cause and effect diagram (fishbone). He has written on quality improvement and the use of quality circles.

Joint Commission on Accreditation for Healthcare Organizations (JCAHO)—An independent, not-for-profit organization dedicated to improving the quality of care in organized health care settings.

Juran, Dr. Joseph M.—Pioneered a statistics-driven philosophy of quality improvement.

Localizing—The process of determining where and when a problem occurs. Obtaining localizing information is important in getting to the root of the problem.

Mission Statement—A statement written by the CEO outlining the purpose and the direction of the organization. The mission statement should be agreed upon by the leadership and be easily measured against a standard.

Multivote—Process used to "weed out" the significant few ideas from a list of many. Usually done after a brainstorming session. One third of the topics are voted on (in public or private) in several stages until a manageable number of topics remain for discussion.

Nominal Group Technique—Process used as a "private" method of determining priorities among a list of brainstorming topics. This technique is best used when the group is not comfortable with each other, or the topics are too sensitive to openly voice an opinion.

Operational Definitions—What something is, and how it should be measured. Operational definitions are crucial to the success of any project.

Pareto chart—A chart based on the Pareto principle: 80 percent of the trouble comes from 20 percent of the problems. The Pareto chart is a histogram that lists out all the problems in rank order.

Peer Review—A critical analysis of job performance for another member of the same profession. Comments should focus on improving the other person's practice, not on faults within the system.

Performance Improvement—The continuous study and adaptation of functions and processes of a health care organization to increase the probability of achieving desired outcomes and to better meet the needs of patients and other users of services.

Performance Improvement team—A multi-disciplinary team formed to evaluate and improve a process that has been identified as needing attention.

Plan-do-check-act Cycle—Otherwise known as the Shewhart cycle.

Prevention Oriented—Central to any prevention effort is a strong planning focus. It is far less costly to fix the problem before it happens.

Process—A goal-directed, interrelated series of actions, events, mechanisms or steps. There may be few or many processes in a given system.

Quality—Both the customer's perception of the product, service or information provided and the supplier's knowledge of customer requirements, variation between customers and applicable standards.

Risk Management—Protecting the organization's financial assets while making the environment safe for patients, visitors and staff.

Run Chart—A run sheet plots data over time. Used to graphically demonstrate a pattern.

Scatter Diagram—A diagram which looks at the relationship between two characteristics. It determines cause(s) for process problems and illustrates what happens to one variable when a second changes. The shape of the resulting plots are indicative of the kind of relationship that exists: positive, negative, or no relationship.

Service-Oriented Strategy—The customer must come first, last, and always.

Shewhart Cycle—The plan-do-check-act cycle for process improvement implementation.

Statistical Process Control (SPC)—A widely used tool to identify common and special cause variations in a process.

Statistical Thinking—Involves: 1. management by facts 2. using an orderly approach, and 3. benchmarking.

Storyboarding—Used to place ideas into categories for all to see. Once in categories, the ideas can be organized and prioritized for further action. Storyboarding is the midway point between brainstorming and the nominal group technique.

Suppliers—People or companies that supply physical needs to physicians, nurses, or payers.

Survey—A common way to collect opinions and demographic data.

System—A collection of processes that work in concert to produce a desired outcome.

Team Approach—To carefully select people for the sole purpose of accomplishing a stated mission. A central theme in Performance Improvement.

Team Building—The act of bringing together a cross section of people who are related to the process in question.

Team Leader—The P.I. team member who has the responsibilities of preparing and conducting the meeting, assessing team progress, and representing the team to management.

Top-down Flow Chart—A chart which lists the major steps in a process along the top with associated substeps listed below. This type of diagram serves two purposes. First, it lists the steps in chronological order. Second, it identifies a step-by-step dependency within the process.

Utilization Management—Evaluation the system to determine over, under and optimum utilization of resources. Resources include manpower, money, and machines.

Variation—Anything that causes the process to waver. Common cause variation is acceptable in a stable process. Special cause variation falls outside the system and must be investigated.

Vision—A long-range target for performance improvement.

Work Flow Diagram—Used to map out traffic patterns within a work area. Use this tool to determine efficiency of the work area relative to the tasks at hand.

Bibliography

Beaudin, C. and Pelletier, L. "Consumer-Based Research: Using Focus Groups as a Method for Evaluating Quality of Care" *Journal of Nursing Care Quality.* 10(3), April 1996 (28-33).

Butler, Joan and Robert J. Parsons. "Hospital perceptions of job satisfaction." *Nursing Management* 20(8): 45-48 (1990).

Consolidated Accreditation Manual for Hospitals. Joint Commission on Accreditation of Healthcare Organizations (JCAHO), Oakbrook Terrace, IL.

Crosby, Phillip B. *Quality is Free: The Art of Making Quality Certain.* New York: McGraw-Hill, 1989.

Deming, Edwards W. *Out of the Crisis.* Cambridge, Mass: Massachusetts Institute of Technology Center for Advanced Engineering Study, 1986.

Ernst & Young Quality Improvement Consulting Group. Total Quality. *An Executive's Guide for the 1990's.* Homewood, IL.: Dow Jones-Irwin, 1990.

Gift, R.G. and Mosel, D. "What is Benchmarking?" *Benchmarking in Health Care: A Collaborative Approach,* New York, NY: American Hospital Association Publishing, 1994.

Ishikawa, Kaoru. *What is Total Quality Control? The Japanese Way.* Englewood Cliffs, NJ: Prentice-Hall, 1985.

Juran, Joseph M. *Juran on Leadership for Quality: An Executive Handbook.* New York: The Free Press, 1979.

Keill, P. and Johnson, T. "Optimizing Performance through Process Improvement" *Journal of Nursing Care Quality,* 9(1), 1994 , 1-9.

Leadership Skills For Performance Improvement: Planning for Quality. Joint Commission on Accreditation of Healthcare Organizations, Oakbrook Terrace, IL, 1995.

Manthey, Marie. "From Mama Management to Team Spirit." *Nursing Management* 21(1): 20-21 (1990).

Merry, Martin D. "Total Quality Management for Physicians: Translating the New Paradigm." *QRB.* 101-105 (1990).

Parisi, Leonard "Selecting Quality Improvement Team Members" *Nursing Quality Connection.* 4(5) March-April, 1995.

Scherkenbach, William W. *The Deming Route to Quality and Productivity.* Rockville, MD: Mercury Press, 1988.

Schmieding, Norma Jean. "Do Head Nurses Include Staff Nurses in Problem Solving?" *Nursing Management* 21(3): 58-60 (1990).

Sholtes, Peter R. *The Team Handbook: How to Use Teams to Improve Quality.* Madison, WI: Joiner Associates, 1989.

Victory, Anne (Sister), et al. "Assessing Nursing Systems Relationships." *Nursing Management.* 21(1): 64Q-64X (1990).

Walton, Mary. *The Deming Management Method.* 3-21. New York: Doss, Mead and Co., 1986.

Williams, Timothy P. and Howe, Rufus S. *Applying Total Quality Management: A Nursing Guide.* National Association of Quality Assurance Professionals and Precept Press, Chicago, 1994.

Young, W, Minnick, A. and Marcantonio, R. "How Wide is the Gap in Defining Quality Care?" *Journal of Nursing Administration,* 26(5), 1996, 15-20.